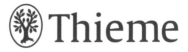

Synopsis of Shoulder Surgery

Uma Srikumaran, MD, MBA, MPH
Associate Professor of Orthopaedic Surgery
Shoulder Fellowship Director
Johns Hopkins School of Medicine;
Chair, Orthopaedic Surgery at Howard County General Hospital
Columbia, Maryland, USA

183 illustrations

Thieme
New York • Stuttgart • Delhi • Rio de Janeiro

Library of Congress Cataloging-in-Publication Data is available with the publisher.

© 2021 Thieme. All rights reserved.

Thieme Publishers New York
333 Seventh Avenue, New York, NY 10001 USA
+1 800 782 3488, customerservice@thieme.com

Georg Thieme Verlag KG
Rüdigerstrasse 14, 70469 Stuttgart, Germany
+49 [0]711 8931 421, customerservice@thieme.de

Thieme Publishers Delhi
A-12, Second Floor, Sector-2, Noida-201301
Uttar Pradesh, India
+91 120 45 566 00, customerservice@thieme.in

Thieme Publishers Rio de Janeiro,
Thieme Publicações Ltda.
Edifício Rodolpho de Paoli, 25º andar
Av. Nilo Peçanha, 50 – Sala 2508,
Rio de Janeiro 20020-906 Brasil
+55 21 3172-2297

Cover design: Thieme Publishing Group
Typesetting by DiTech Process Solutions, India

Printed in USA by King Printing Company, Inc.

5 4 3 2 1

ISBN 978-1-68420-080-1

Also available as an e-book:
eISBN 978-1-68420-081-8

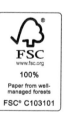

FSC
www.fsc.org
100%
Paper from well-managed forests
FSC® C103101

To all the students, residents, and fellows who have taught me so much.

Uma Srikumaran

Contents

Contents

Contents

Contents

Preface

Synopsis of Shoulder Surgery presents a succinct summary of a comprehensive range of shoulder conditions in an easy-to-understand format.

Based on the underlying type of pathology, chapters have been organized to cover topics like epidemiology, pathophysiology, anatomy, presentation, imaging, and both nonoperative and surgical treatment.

As information is presented in a bulleted outline format, readers can easily find areas of interest within larger subject areas. While the book has been organized in a logical format for those interested in reading it from start to finish, the text can also serve as a quick reference guide for a particular topic of interest. This book will be useful for students, orthopaedic surgeons-in-training, frontline practitioners, including allied health professionals, and nonoperative specialists.

I hope this book will be an invaluable resource for the readers that will help them gain a broad understanding of the shoulder, its common pathologies, and how they are managed.

Uma Srikumaran, MD, MBA, MPH

Contributors

Clayton Alexander, MD
Orthopaedic Hand Surgeon
The Shoulder, Elbow, Wrist, and Hand Center
Division of the Orthopaedic Specialty Hospital
Mercy Medical Center
Baltimore, Maryland, USA

Matthew Baker, MD
Orthopaedic Surgeon
Department of Orthopaedics
Southeast Orthopaedics and Sports Medicine
Cape Girardeau, Missouri, USA

Ankit Bansal, MD
Orthopaedic Surgeon
Department of Orthopaedic Surgery
Mercy Health Physicians
Cincinnati, Ohio, USA

Matthew Binkley, MD
Clinical Assistant Professor
Shoulder and Elbow Surgery Specialist
Department of Orthopaedics and
    Sports Medicine
University at Buffalo
Buffalo, New York, USA

Alexander Bitzer, MD
Sports Medicine and Shoulder/Elbow Surgeon
Department of Orthopaedic Surgery
Johns Hopkins Hospital
Baltimore, Maryland, USA

Joseph Ferraro, MD
Orthopaedic Surgery Resident
Department of Orthopaedics and
    Sports Medicine
University at Buffalo
Buffalo, New York, USA

Nickolas G. Garbis, MD, FAAOS
Associate Professor
Department of Orthopaedic Surgery and
    Rehabilitation
Loyola University Medical Center
Maywood, Illinois, USA

Eric G. Huish Jr, DO
Orthopaedic Surgeon
Department of Orthopaedic Surgery
San Joaquin General Hospital
French Camp, California, USA

Kelly G. Kilcoyne, MD
Associate Professor
Uniformed Services University of the
    Health Sciences
Shoulder and Elbow Surgery Specialist
Department of Orthopaedics
Walter Reed National Military Medical Center
Bethesda, Maryland, USA

Alexander E. Loeb, MD
Resident
Department of Orthopaedics
John Hopkins Medicine
Baltimore, Maryland, USA

Suresh K. Nayar, MD
Resident
Department of Orthopaedics
John Hopkins Medicine
Baltimore, Maryland, USA

Ian S. Patten, MD, MPH
Resident
Department of Orthopaedic Surgery
John Hopkins Medicine
Baltimore, Maryland, USA

Paul S. Ragusa, DO
Orthopaedic Surgeon
Orthopedic Surgery and Sports Medicine of
    New York
Yonkers, New York, USA

Andrew Schneider, MD
Resident Physician
Department of Orthopaedic Surgery
Loyola University Medical Center
Maywood, Illinois, USA

Uma Srikumaran, MD, MBA, MPH
Associate Professor of Orthopaedic Surgery
Shoulder Fellowship Director
Johns Hopkins School of Medicine;
Chair, Orthopaedic Surgery at Howard County
    General Hospital
Columbia, Maryland, USA

Scott Wagner, MD
Assistant Professor
Department of Orthopaedics
Walter Reed National Military Medical Center
Uniformed Services University of the
    Health Sciences
Bethesda, Maryland, USA

Diana Zhu, MD
Resident Physician
Department of Orthopaedics
John Hopkins Medicine
Baltimore, Maryland, USA

1 Shoulder Anatomy

Nickolas G. Garbis

Summary

The chapter is intended to be a high-level overview of shoulder anatomy and a quick reference for trainees and surgeons.

Keywords: Shoulder, anatomy, muscles, nerves, tendons

I. General introduction

Λ. Complex joint

B. Helps position the arm in space

C. Essential in allowing us to interact with the environment

D. Connects the axial skeleton to the upper extremity.

II. Bones and joints

A. Shoulder girdle is composed of four bones:

    1. Sternum

    2. Clavicle

    3. Scapula

    4. Humerus.

B. Three major articulations:

    1. Sternoclavicular (SC) joint

    2. Acromioclavicular (AC) joint

    3. Glenohumeral (GH) joint.

C. Other articulations and spaces:

    1. Subacromial space

    2. Scapulothoracic bursa.

III. Sternum

A. Connection point of the appendicular skeleton to the axial skeleton

B. Bone is composed of three parts:

    1. Manubrium

    2. Body

    3. Xiphoid process.

C. Sternal notch is a depression between the two SC joints

D. SC joints are shallow notches at the superolateral corners of the manubrium (▶ **Fig. 1.1**)

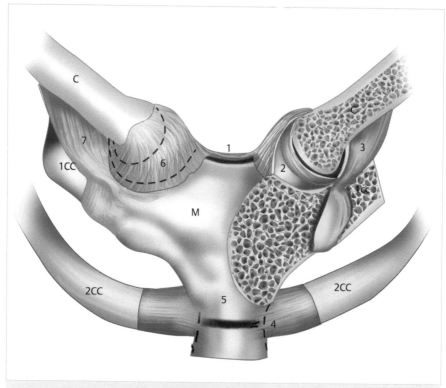

Fig. 1.1 Diagram of the sternoclavicular (SC) joint. 1CC, first costal cartilage (ossified); 2CC, second costal cartilage; M, manubrium; 1, interclavicular ligament; 2, articular disc; 3, costoclavicular ligament (posterior lamina); 4, sternocostal joint; 5, manubriosternal joint; 6, anterior sternoclavicular ligament; 7, costoclavicular ligament (anterior lamina).

E. The body and manubrium serve as insertion points for the costal cartilages of ribs 1–7

F. Important to understand role of SC articulation in shoulder biomechanics.

IV. Clavicle

A. Bone that spans from the sternum to the acromion

B. Flat near the lateral third but becomes more convex medially

C. Begins ossifying at 5 weeks in utero

D. The medial epiphysis of the clavicle is the last to fuse at approximately 23–25 years of life

E. The size of the bone changes in cross section at different points:

    1. 23 mm × 22 mm at the sternal end

    2. 12 mm × 12 mm at the diaphysis

    3. 21 mm × 11 mm at the lateral end.

F. The coracoclavicular and AC ligaments stabilize the clavicle (▶ **Fig. 1.2**):

1. The conoid and trapezoid ligaments provide the primary restraint in the craniocaudal direction

2. The AC ligaments provide restraint in the anteroposterior direction.

G. Biomechanically, the clavicle acts as a strut to support the arm for activities performed away from the body

H. Serves as protection for the underlying neurovascular structures:

1. Can provide mechanical advantage for the myofascial sleeve around it.

V. Scapula

A. Triangular flat bone

B. Multiple prominences

C. Point of fixation for several upper extremity muscles

D. Has a curved contour to articulate with the rib cage

E. The spine of the scapula divides the supraspinatus and infraspinatus fossae (▶ **Fig. 1.3**)

F. The coracoid process is an anterior projection and an important surgical landmark:

1. Sometimes called "the lighthouse" of the shoulder

2. The coracobrachialis and short head of the biceps conjoined tendon have their origin in the coracoid

3. The pectoralis minor inserts on the medial aspect of the coracoid (▶ **Fig. 1.4**)

4. The coracoacromial and coracoclavicular ligaments also attach to the coracoid.

G. The acromion process is usually easily palpable in the subcutaneous tissue at the lateral aspect of the scapula:

1. Connects the clavicle to the scapula at the AC joint

2. Serves as the origin of the deltoid muscle.

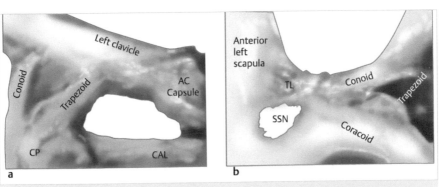

Fig. 1.2 Gross anatomy of the coracoclavicular ligaments. (a) Anterior view. (b) Anterior medial view. CP, coracoid process; TL, transverse ligament; SSN, suprascapular nerve; CAL, coracoacromial ligament.

3

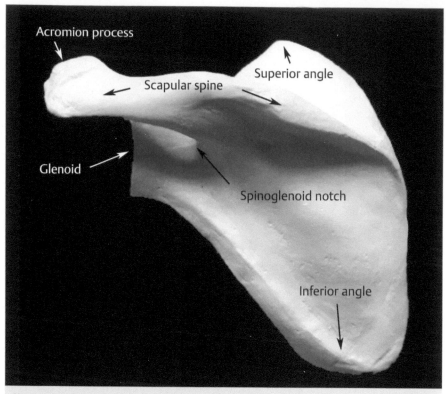

Fig. 1.3 Posterior view of a left scapula.

H. The scapula widens laterally into the glenoid neck and glenoid fossa:
1. Glenoid anatomy is variable but usually version will range from 9.5 degrees of anteversion to 10.5 degrees of retroversion
2. The mean inclination of the glenoid is usually 4 degrees of superior tilt
3. Size usually 27.8 mm by 37.5 mm in men and 23.6 mm by 32.6 mm in women.

VI. Humerus

A. Extension of the shoulder joint that allows positioning of the arm in space
B. The humeral head articulates with the glenoid:
1. The average radius of curvature is 24 mm in the coronal plane
2. The average thickness has been reported to be 19 mm
3. The average articular surface diameter is 43 mm.

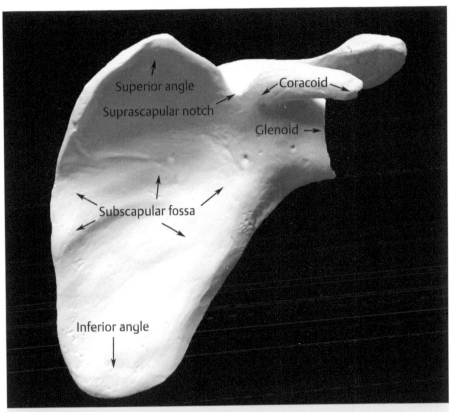

Fig. 1.4 Anterior view of a left scapula.

C. The greater and lesser tuberosities are the attachment points of the rotator cuff (▶**Fig. 1.5**):

1. Subscapularis attaches to the lesser tuberosity
2. Supraspinatus, infraspinatus, and teres minor attach to the greater tuberosity
3. The biceps groove is between the tuberosities, and can be a useful landmark during surgery.

D. Retroversion of the proximal humerus is variable and can be anywhere from 10 to 5 degrees. It averages approximately 30 degrees of retroversion.

VII. Sternoclavicular joint

A. Joint between medial end of the clavicle and the superolateral aspect of the sternum

B. Has been described as both a ball and socket and a saddle joint

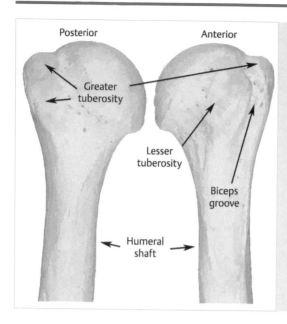

Fig. 1.5 Posterior and anterior views of the proximal humerus demonstrating the tuberosities and the bicipital groove.

C. The first costal cartilage is at the inferior aspect of the SC joint

D. Only bony connection of the upper extremity to the axial skeleton

E. Thickenings of the capsule serve to provide ligamentous restraint

1. The posterior SC ligament serves as primary restraint for the SC joint

2. The medial end of the clavicle is attached to the first rib with the costoclavicular ligament which helps restrict superior migration

3. There is an articular disc in the SC joint that attaches superiorly and inferiorly.

F. The SC joint moves approximately 30–35 degrees in elevation and 35 degrees in flexion/extension

G. Most of the motion in the SC joint occurs in the first 90 degrees of elevation.

VIII. Acromioclavicular (AC) joint

A. The AC joint is the articulation between the medial end of the acromion and the lateral end of the clavicle

B. The ends of the clavicle and the acromion at the AC joint are both covered in fibrocartilage (▶Fig. 1.6):

1. There is also a meniscoid articular disc that covers mostly the superior portion of the joint.

C. The angle of the AC joint can be variable and should be considered during surgical planning

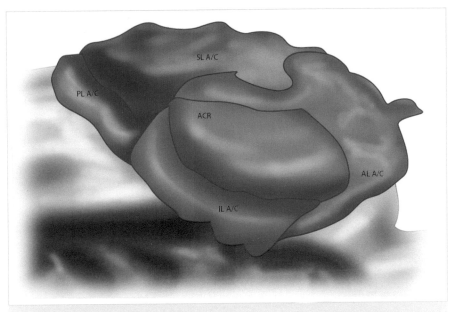

Fig. 1.6 Left shoulder: acromial side of the AC joint. The entire capsule, detached from the clavicular side, is still attached at the acromial side, making the acromioclavicular ligaments visible. ACR, acromion, articular side; AL A/C, anterior acromioclavicular ligament; IL A/C, inferior acromioclavicular ligament; PL A/C, posterior acromioclavicular ligament; SL A/C, superior acromioclavicular ligament.

D. The AC ligament provides most of the anterior and posterior stability

E. The coracoclavicular ligaments provide most of the vertical stability and help maintain the relationship between the clavicle and the coracoid:

   1. Composed of the trapezoid (anterolateral) and conoid (posteromedial) ligaments.

IX. Glenohumeral joint

A. Ball and socket or "ball on golf tee" joint that serves as the articulation between the humerus and the scapula (▶ Fig. 1.7)

B. Allows a significant amount of mobility to help position the arm in space:

   1. Several dynamic and static restraints to motion

   2. Only a small portion of the humeral head surface contacts the glenoid at any given point.

C. The glenoid fossa is surrounded by a fibrocartilaginous labrum that provides stability and deepens the articular surface

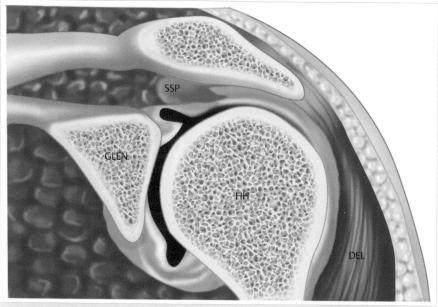

Fig. 1.7 Left shoulder, frontal view. DEL, deltoid; GLEN, glenoid; HH, humeral head; SSP, supraspinatus.

D. The labrum is an attachment point for the joint capsule, glenohumeral ligaments, and long head of the biceps tendon

E. Capsulolabral tears can allow for increased glenohumeral translation

F. Bone loss at the glenoid can decrease the size of the articular surface and lead to increased instability

G. Several named thickenings of the joint capsule provide static restraint to the glenohumeral joint (▶ **Fig. 1.8**)

H. The inferior glenohumeral ligament is analogous to a hammock at the inferior aspect of the shoulder joint:

   1. Anterior band (AIGHL)

   2. Posterior band (PIGHL)

   3. Axillary pouch (AxIGHL)

   4. With the arm in abduction, further external rotation will tighten the ligament and keep the humeral head centered on the glenoid.

I. The middle glenohumeral ligament (MGHL) (▶ **Fig. 1.9**) limits external rotation with the arm at the side:

   1. The MGHL usually originates from the upper anterior glenoid, runs deep to the subscapularis, and inserts on the lesser tuberosity

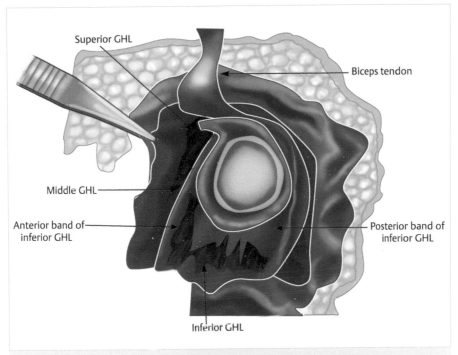

Fig. 1.8 Left cadaveric shoulder demonstrating labrum and intra-articular ligaments. GHL, glenohumeral ligament.

2. There are several anatomic variants of the MGHL:
   a. A sublabral foramen is present in 12% of cases
   b. A cord-like MGHL is present in 18% of cases
   c. A Buford complex is found in 1–2% of cases:
      i. Anterior superior labrum is absent and a cord-like MGHL originates from the superior labrum.

J. The superior glenohumeral ligament (SGHL) limits external rotation and inferior translation:
   1. Originates anterior to the biceps at the supraglenoid tubercle, but this origin can be variable.

K. The posterior capsule can become pathologically thickened and limit posterior translation and adduction across the body

L. The coracoacromial ligament, acromion, and coracoid all serve as static stabilizers to prevent superior migration of the humeral head

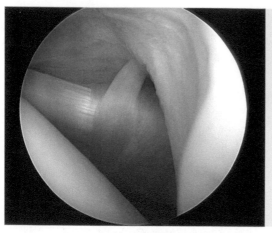

Fig. 1.9 Arthroscopic image of the middle glenohumeral ligament (MGHL) coming off at 90 degrees angle to the subscapularis tendon. Patient is in the beach chair position (image taken from the posterior portal).

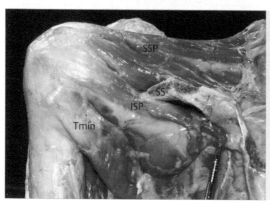

Fig. 1.10 Posterior view of the shoulder demonstrating the rotator cuff musculature. SSP, supraspinatus; SS, scapular spine; ISP, infraspinatus; Tmin, teres minor.

M. The glenohumeral joint is stabilized through the midrange of motion by dynamic stabilizers:

1. These consist of the rotator cuff and periscapular muscles (▶ **Fig. 1.10** and ▶ **Fig. 1.11**)

2. The long head of the biceps may assist in depressing the humeral head, but its role has been debated

3. The rotator cuff provides compression of the humeral head into the glenoid fossa, which further increases stability.

X. Subacromial space

A. The space between the rotator cuff and the undersurface of the acromion and deltoid

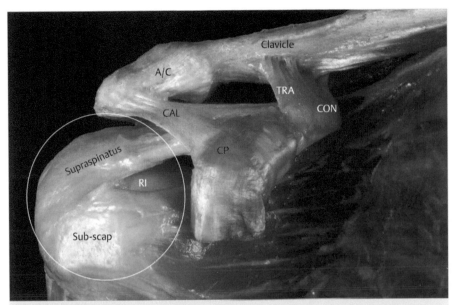

Fig. 1.11 Anterior view of the shoulder demonstrating relationship of subscapularis to the supraspinatus. RI, rotator interval; CP, coracoid process; A/C, acromioclavicular ligaments; CAL, coracoacromial ligament; TRA, trapezoid; CON, conoid.

B. Several structures can be assessed (▶ **Fig. 1.12**):

1. Rotator cuff

2. CA ligament

3. AC joint

4. Acromion

5. Biceps.

C. Can describe morphology of acromion as Type 1 (flat), Type II (curved), or Type III (hooked) (▶ **Fig. 1.13**).

XI. Scapulothoracic bursa

A. Several bursae that glide over the ribcage

B. Two major bursae:

1. Scapulothoracic bursa

2. Subscapularis bursa.

C. Four minor bursae are not always identifiable, and usually present only in cases of pathologic scapulothoracic articulation (▶ **Fig. 1.14**).

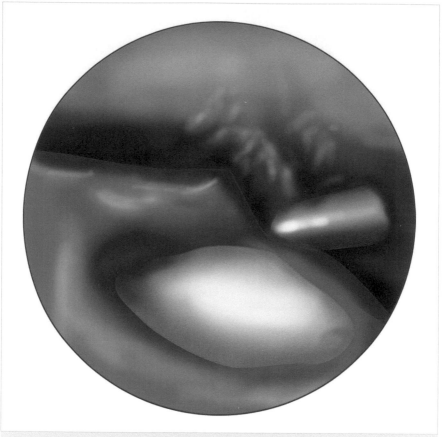

Fig. 1.12 View of the right subacromial space from a posterior portal in beach chair position demonstrating a supraspinatus tear.

XII. Muscles

A. There are several muscles that act around the shoulder:

    1. It can be helpful to group into regions or think of them based on origin or insertion

    2. The muscles that act on the shoulder usually originate from the scapula itself, the ribs and chest wall, or the spinous processes

    3. See ▶ Table 1.1 for more detail.

XIII. Neurovascular anatomy

A. Important to understand the anatomy of the brachial plexus

    1. Composed of C5–T1 nerve roots

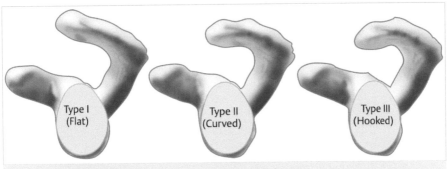

Fig. 1.13 Enface view of the scapula demonstrating acromial morphology.

2. Roots, trunks, divisions, cords, and branches (▶ **Fig. 1.15**)
3. Four preclavicular branches which come from rami and trunks:
   a. Dorsal scapular nerve
   b. Long thoracic nerve
   c. Suprascapular nerve
   d. Nerve to subclavius.

B. Vascular anatomy of the axillary artery branches is organized by its relationship to the pectoralis minor:
   1. Axillary artery is a continuation of the subclavian artery
   2. The subclavian artery comes off the brachiocephalic trunk on the right and aorta on the left
   3. It becomes the axillary artery at the lateral aspect of the first rib
   4. Supreme thoracic artery is the only axillary artery branch that originates medial to pectoralis minor
   5. Deep to the pectoralis minor, it gives off branches to the thoracoacromial artery and the lateral thoracic arteries:
      a. Thoracoacromial has four branches:
         i. Acromial
         ii. Clavicular
         iii. Pectoral
         iv. Deltoid.
   6. Lateral to the pectoralis minor, it branches into the posterior circumflex, anterior circumflex, and subscapular arteries.

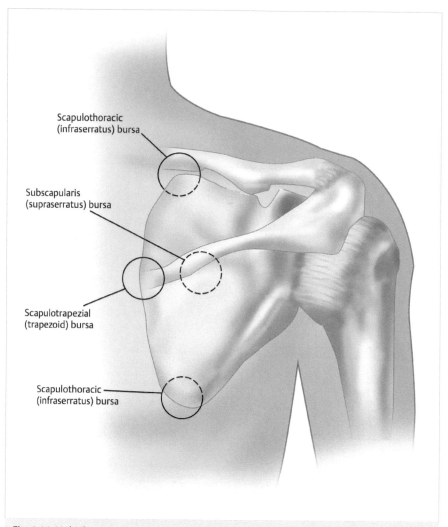

Scapulothoracic
(infraserratus) bursa

Subscapularis
(supraserratus) bursa

Scapulotrapezial
(trapezoid) bursa

Scapulothoracic
(infraserratus) bursa

Fig. 1.14 Multiple named bursae around the shoulder, anteroposterior (AP) view.

Table 1.1 Muscle origins, insertions, and innervations about the shoulder

Muscle	Origin	Insertion	Function	Innervation
Pectoralis minor	Ribs three to five	Medial aspect of the coracoid	Protracts scapula	Medial pectoral nerve
Pectoralis major	Sternum, clavicle, ribs	Lateral aspect of the bicipital groove	Adducts and internally rotates arm	Medial and lateral pectoral nerves
Latissimus dorsi	Spinous processes of thoracolumbar spine and ilium	Medial aspect of the bicipital groove	Extends, adducts, internally rotates humerus	Dorsal scapular nerve
Trapezius	Spinous processes C7–C12	Posterior surface lateral third clavicle, acromion, scapular spine	Rotates scapula	Spinal accessory nerve (cranial nerve XI)
Rhomboid major	Spinous processes T2–T5	Medial border scapula	Adducts scapula	Dorsal scapular nerve
Rhomboid minor	Spinous processes C7–T1	Medial aspect of scapular spine	Adducts scapula	Dorsal scapular nerve
Levator scapulae	Transverse processes C1–C4	Superomedial scapula	Move scapula cephalad and rotate	C3 and C4
Subclavius	First rib	Inferior clavicle	Moves clavicle caudally	Upper trunk brachial plexus
Serratus anterior	First through ninth rib	Ventral medial surface of scapula	Holds scapula against chest wall	Long thoracic nerve
Deltoid	Lateral aspect clavicle, acromion, and scapular spine	Deltoid tuberosity of humerus	Abducts arm	Axillary nerve
Teres major	Inferior scapula	Medial aspect bicipital groove	Adducts, internally rotates, extends arm	Lower subscapular nerve
Subscapularis	Ventral scapula	Lesser tuberosity	Internally rotates arm	Upper and lower subscapular nerves
Supraspinatus	Supraspinous fossa	Greater tuberosity	Abducts and internally rotates arm	Suprascapular nerve
Infraspinatus	Infraspinous fossa	Greater tuberosity	Externally rotates arm	Suprascapular nerve
Teres minor	Dorsolateral scapula	Greater tuberosity	Externally rotates arm	Axillary nerve
Biceps brachii	Supraglenoid tubercle (long head) and coracoid (short head)	Radial tuberosity	Flex and supinate elbow	Musculocutaneous nerve

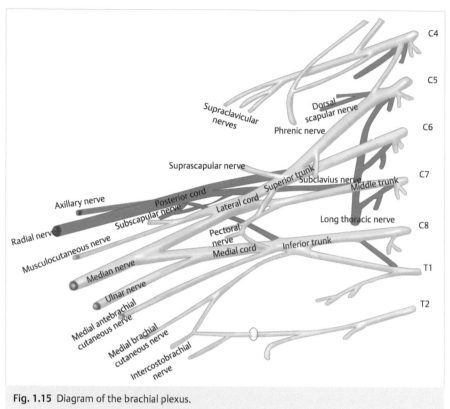

Fig. 1.15 Diagram of the brachial plexus.

Suggested Readings

Hoppenfeld S, de Boer P, Buckley R. The shoulder. In: Surgical Exposures in Orthopaedics: The Anatomic Approach. Philadelphia, PA: Lippincott Williams & amp; Wilkins; 2009

Jobe CM, Phipatanakul WP, Petkovic D. Gross anatomy of the shoulder In: Rockwood CA et al, eds. Rockwood and Matsen's The Shoulder. Philadelphia, PA: Elsevier; 2017

O'Brien SJ et al. Developmental anatomy of the shoulder and anatomy of the glenohumeral joint. In: Rockwood CA et al, eds. Rockwood and Matsen's The Shoulder. Philadelphia, PA: Elsevier; 2017

2 Complications in Shoulder Arthroscopy

Clayton Alexander and Uma Srikumaran

Summary

Arthroscopic shoulder surgery complications are considered rare occurrences. However, there have been reports in the literature of complication rates as high as 10.6%. It is imperative to evaluate the incidence, severity, and prevention of these complications to improve surgical outcomes. Common complications reported after arthroscopic shoulder surgery are peripheral nerve injury, infections, arthrofibrosis, and thromboembolic events. Careful patient selection, surgical diligence, and extensive knowledge of the shoulder anatomy can prevent these complications.

Keywords: Shoulder arthroscopy, complications, nerve injury, arthrofibrosis, infection

I. Incidence and patient risk factors

A. Arthroscopic shoulder complications are less prevalent than open shoulder procedures[1]

B. Complication rates following arthroscopic shoulder procedures range from 1.0 to 10.6%:[2,7]

    1. Wide range due to definition of complications and length of follow-up.

C. Common complications include:[8]

    1. Arthrofibrosis/stiffness

    2. Infections

    3. Deep vein thrombosis/pulmonary embolism (DVT/PE)

    4. Peripheral nerve injury.

D. Patient risk factors:[1]

    1. Age > 80 years

    2. Body mass index (BMI) > 35

    3. Functionally dependent status

    4. American Society of Anesthesiology > 2 (Class III or IV)

    5. Congestive heart failure

    6. History of disseminated cancer

    7. Open wound at time of surgery.

II. Patient positioning

No proven difference in complication rates between lateral decubitus and beach chair positions.[8]

A. Lateral decubitus (▶ **Fig. 2.1**):

    1. Theoretical benefits:

        a. Increased visualization and access

        b. Lower risk of hypotension, bradycardia, and cerebral hypoperfusion.

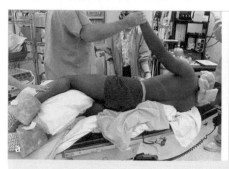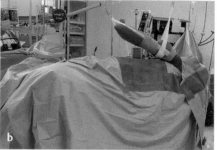

Fig. 2.1 (a, b) Patient is in the lateral decubitus position and the surgical arm is held in an abducted position.[8]

    2. Potential complications:

        a. Neuropraxia from arm traction (10–30%)

        b. Higher rate of thromboembolic events

        c. Increased risk of injury to axillary and musculocutaneous nerves when placing anteroinferior portal.[9]

B. Beach chair (▶ **Fig. 2.2**):

    1. Theoretical benefits:

        a. Better anatomic orientation

        b. Easier to convert to open procedure

        c. Regional anesthesia is better tolerated than with lateral positions

        d. Decreased risk of neuropathies

        e. Decreased surgical time.

    2. Potential hypoperfusion complications:

        a. Cerebral hypoperfusion:

            i. Can be reduced with use of regional anesthesia instead of general anesthesia.

        b. Neuropraxia from head and neck malpositioning.[10]

III. Anatomy and nerve injury

Iatrogenic nerve injuries are common due to proximity of the standard portals to the nerves[8] and lack of awareness of anatomical variations of the nerves.[11]

A. Axillary nerve:

    1. Distance of axillary nerve from:[8]

        a. Coracoid process tip: 3.56 ± 0.51 cm (immediately before entering the quadrangular space)

        b. Posterolateral acromion: 7.46 ± 0.99 cm

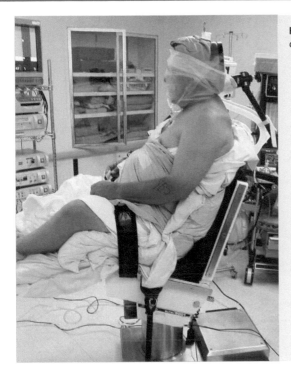

Fig. 2.2 Patient is in the beach chair position preoperatively.[8]

    c.   Deltoid insertion: 6.7 ± 0.47 cm

    d.   Upper border of deltoid origin:

        i.   Anterior: 4.94 ± 0.8 6 cm

        ii.   Middle: 5.14 ± 0.90 cm

        iii.   Posterior: 5.44 ± 0.95 cm.

2.   Axillary nerve comes closest to capsule at 5:30–6:30 o'clock positions on the glenoid with the closest distance measuring 10–25 mm away[12]

3.   Standard posterior portal placement is usually a minimum of 2–3 cm from the axillary nerve:

    a.   Placement is also 2 cm medial and 2 cm inferior to the posterolateral corner of the acromion.

4.   Lateral working portals placed in the "safe zone" (located within 3 cm of the lateral border of the acromion) avoid the axillary nerve

5.   Anterior portals, particularly anteroinferior portals, are at greater risk of neurovascular injury than posterior portals:

    a.   Increasing risk of axillary nerve injury with inferior placement

    b.   Placement of anterior portal lateral to the coracoid through the rotator interval is safe.

6. Specific arthroscopic procedures at higher risk of axillary nerve injury:

    a. Glenohumeral capsular release:

        i. Through anteroinferior or posteroinferior axillary pouch and recesses places the nerve at risk of injury.

    b. Thermal capsulorrhaphy

    c. Arthroscopic stabilization:

        i. Capsulolabral sutures of anteroinferior band of the inferior glenohumeral ligament have particular risk

        ii. Sutures placed within 1 cm of the anterior glenoid rim are relatively safe.

    d. Arthroscopic axillary nerve release

    e. Arthroscopic Latarjet:

        i. Close proximity of surgical instruments to axillary nerves.[8]

B. Musculocutaneous nerve:

    1. At risk with anterior working portal (▶ **Fig. 2.3**):

    a. Standard placement of portal is midway between anterolateral corner of the acromion and coracoid

    b. More inferior or medial placement of portal increases chances of injury

    c. Less risk of injury with placement under direct visualization.[8]

C. Suprascapular nerve:

    1. Unique anatomy of nerve makes it susceptible to injury during various open and arthroscopic shoulder procedures:[8]

    a. Transglenoid drilling for instability:

        i. Anchors have shown to decrease this risk.

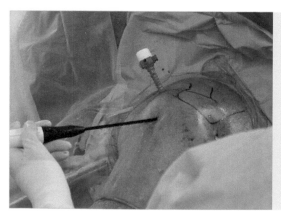

Fig. 2.3 Anterior arthroscopic working portal is placed midway between the coracoid and anterolateral acromion.[8]

b. Aggressive mobilization of retracted rotator cuff tear:

    i. Risk is minimized by staying within 2 cm of superior glenoid rim.

c. Arthroscopic decompression of suprascapular and spinoglenoid notches increases the vulnerability of the nerve to injury

d. Arthroscopic transglenoid Bankart repair:[13]

    i. Usually transient injuries.

IV. Infection

A. Deep infection after arthroscopic shoulder procedure is rare but can be devastating:

  1. Overall rate ranges from 0 to 3.4%.[7,14,15]

B. Risk for infection increases drastically when converted to open procedure

C. Risk factors for perioperative infection following arthroscopic shoulder procedure are:

  1. Diabetes mellitus

  2. Smoking

  3. Obesity

  4. Peripheral vascular disease

  5. Immunocompromised

  6. History of prior surgery

  7. Prior joint aspiration or injection.

D. *Propionibacterium acnes* has predilection for postoperative shoulder infection:

  1. Gram positive bacillus

  2. Can take up to 2 weeks to grow in culture

  3. Mildly virulent with often benign initial presentation

  4. Usually no systemic symptoms, no laboratory abnormalities, and minimal to no local reaction

  5. Usually penicillin (PCN) sensitive

  6. Vigilance is required to identify this infection in a timely manner.[8]

E. Efficacy of surgical preparation solutions in removing bacteria from shoulder region:[16]

  1. ChloraPrep is more effective than DuraPrep and povidone-iodine

  2. DuraPrep is more effective than povidone-iodine

  3. Antibiotic prophylaxis can drastically reduce infection rates following arthroscopic shoulder procedures.[14]

F. Deep infection is treated successfully with surgical debridement and antibiotic therapy.[8]

V. Venous thromboembolic events

A. Venous thromboembolic events (VTE) after arthroscopic shoulder surgery are rare:

    1. Overall pulmonary embolism rate: 0.01%

    2. Overall DVT rate: <0.01%.

B. Thromboprophylaxis is not particularly useful in preventing VTE after arthroscopic shoulder procedures.[17]

VI. Athrofibrosis and stiffness

A. Postarthroscopic athrofibrosis:

    1. Rate of postarthroscopic arthrofibrosis in the shoulder: 1–2.8%

    2. Classic arthrofibrosis is intra-articular adhesions in the glenohumeral joint:

        a. May be present with extra-articular adhesions in multiple periarticular locations.

    3. General comorbid associations:

        a. Diabetes

        b. History of keloid formation.

    4. Treated initially with physical therapy:

        a. Postsurgical stiffness is more resistant than primary adhesive capsulitis to conservative measures

        b. Surgical interventions such as capsular release are highly successful.[18]

B. Arthroscopic rotator cuff repair (aRCR):

    1. High incidence of stiffness after aRCR: 2.3–8.7%[5,18]

    2. Stiffness is one of the most common complications after primary aRCR:

        a. Stiffness complication rate is 8.7% compared to overall complication rate of 10.6%

        b. Stiffness can be defined as more than 90 postoperative days with:

            i. Passive external rotation less than 10 degrees with arm at the side

            ii. Passive external rotation less than 30 degrees with arm at 90 degrees of abduction

            iii. Passive forward elevation less than 100 degrees.

        c. Stiffness in most patients is treated successfully with physical therapy:

            i. Arthroscopic release can be performed if nonoperative treatments fail.[5]

    3. Risk factors for stiffness after aRCR:[18]

        a. Prolonged immobilization

        b. Noncompliance with physical therapy

        c. Over-tightening of repair

      d.   Glenohumeral osteoarthritis

      e.   Concomitant calcific tendonitis

      f.   History of adhesive capsulitis

      g.   Single tendon repair or repair of partial, articular-sided tear.

4.   Protective factors for postoperative stiffness in the setting of aRCR:[18,19]

      a.   Larger tears

      b.   Multitendon tears

      c.   Concomitant coracoplasty.

C.   Arthroscopic labral repair:

1.   Stiffness is one of the most common complications after superior labrum from anterior to posterior (SLAP) tear repair[20]

2.   Lack of high-quality evidence in the literature to guide successful treatment of stiffness after arthroscopic SLAP lesion repair:[20,21]

      a.   Increased likelihood of unsuccessful conservative treatment

      b.   Recurrent stiffness after operative treatment for postoperative stiffness is also common.

References

1. Rubenstein WJ, Pean CA, Colvin AC. Shoulder arthroscopy in adults 60 or older: risk factors that correlate with postoperative complications in the first 30 days. Arthroscopy 2017;33(1):49–54

2. Shields E, Thirukumaran C, Thorsness R, Noyes K, Voloshin I. An analysis of adult patient risk factors and complications within 30 days after arthroscopic shoulder surgery. Arthroscopy 2015;31(5):807–815

3. Berjano P, González BG, Olmedo JF, Perez-España LA, Munilla MG. Complications in arthroscopic shoulder surgery. Arthroscopy 1998;14(8):785–788

4. Marecek GS, Saltzman MD. Complications in shoulder arthroscopy. Orthopedics 2010;33(7):492–497

5. Brislin KJ, Field LD, Savoie FH III. Complications after arthroscopic rotator cuff repair. Arthroscopy 2007;23(2):124–128

6. Small NC; Committee on Complications of the Arthroscopy Association of North America. Complications in arthroscopy: the knee and other joints. Arthroscopy 1986;2(4):253–258

7. Weber SC, Abrams JS, Nottage WM. Complications associated with arthroscopic shoulder surgery. Arthroscopy 2002;18(2, Suppl 1):88–95

8. Moen TC, Rudolph GH, Caswell K. Espinoza C, Burkhead WZ Jr, Krishnan SG. Complications of shoulder arthroscopy. J Am Acad Orthop Surg 2014;22(7):410–419

9. Jinnah AH, Mannava S, Plate JF, Stone AV, Freehill MT. Basic shoulder arthroscopy: lateral decubitus patient positioning. Arthrosc Tech 2016;5(5):e1069–e1075

10. Mannava S, Jinnah AH, Plate JF, Stone AV, Tuohy CJ, Freehill MT. Basic shoulder arthroscopy: beach chair patient positioning. Arthrosc Tech 2016;5(4):e731 e735

11. Gurushantappa PK, Kuppasad S. Anatomy of axillary nerve and its clinical importance: a cadaveric study. J Clin Diagn Res 2015;9(3):AC13–AC17

12. Scully WF, Wilson DJ, Parada SA, Arrington ED. Iatrogenic nerve injuries in shoulder surgery. J Am Acad Orthop Surg 2013;21(12):717–726

13. Hayashida K, Yoneda M, Nakagawa S, Okamura K, Fukushima S. Arthroscopic Bankart suture repair for traumatic anterior shoulder instability: analysis of the causes of a recurrence. Arthroscopy 1998;14(3):295–301

14. Randelli P, Castagna A, Cabitza F, Cabitza P, Arrigoni P, Denti M. Infectious and thromboembolic complications of arthroscopic shoulder surgery. J Shoulder Elbow Surg 2010;19(1):97–101

15. Marrero LG, Nelman KR, Nottage WM. Long-term follow-up of arthroscopic rotator cuff repair. Arthroscopy 2011;27(7):885–888

16. Saltzman MD, Nuber GW, Gryzlo SM, Marecek GS, Koh JL. Efficacy of surgical preparation solutions in shoulder surgery. J Bone Joint Surg Am 2009;91(8):1949–1953

17. Jameson SS, James P, Howcroft DW, et al. Venous thromboembolic events are rare after shoulder surgery: analysis of a national database. J Shoulder Elbow Surg 2011;20(5):764–770

18. Vezeridis PS, Goel DP, Shah AA, Sung SY, Warner JJ. Postarthroscopic arthrofibrosis of the shoulder. Sports Med Arthrosc Rev 2010;18(3):198–206

19. Huberty DP, Schoolfield JD, Brady PC, Vadala AP, Arrigoni P, Burkhart SS. Incidence and treatment of post-operative stiffness following arthroscopic rotator cuff repair. Arthroscopy 2009;25(8):880–890

20. Brockmeier SF, Voos JE, Williams RJ, Altchek DW, Cordasco FA, Allen AA; Hospital for Special Surgery Sports Medicine and Shoulder Service. Outcomes after arthroscopic repair of type-II SLAP lesions. J Bone Joint Surg Am 2009;91(7):1595–1603

21. Katz LM, Hsu S, Miller SL, et al. Poor outcomes after SLAP repair: descriptive analysis and prognosis. Arthroscopy 2009;25(8):849–855

3 Surgical Approaches to the Shoulder

Nickolas G. Garbis and Diana Zhu

Summary

There are a few basic open approaches that can be used for shoulder surgery. Selecting the appropriate approach can help facilitate operative goals.

Keywords: Shoulder, approach, surgical technique, deltopectoral

I. General introduction

A. As comfort increases with arthroscopic techniques, less shoulder surgery is being performed through open approaches

B. Important to understand anatomy and open approaches to the shoulder.

II. Deltopectoral approach

A. One of the more common anterior approaches to the shoulder

B. Wide utility for a variety of different procedures

C. Internervous plane between the pectoralis major (medial and lateral pectoral nerves) and the deltoid (axillary nerve)

D. Exposes the coracoid, subscapularis, anterior humerus, biceps, and glenoid

E. Can be used as an extensile approach and combined with an anterolateral approach to the humerus (▶ Fig. 3.1)

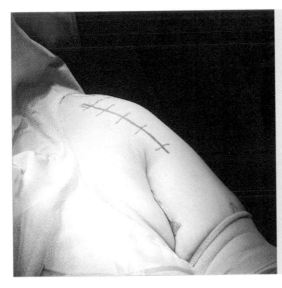

Fig. 3.1 Incision for a deltopectoral approach to the shoulder. Incision is starting at the coracoid and extending toward the pectoralis insertion on the humerus.

F. Operating room setup:
1. Usually performed in the semi-sitting (Beach chair) or supine position
2. Can be performed with patient in lateral position but may be more uncomfortable for surgeon
3. May use a commercial head holder or positioning device to assist with positioning (▶ Fig. 3.2):
    a. These can improve access to posterior shoulder for portal placement
    b. They help maintain cervical spine in neutral alignment
    c. They can assist with dislocation of the humeral head during arthroplasty.
4. A more upright position can lead to a flatter surgeon hand position during arthroscopy procedures
5. A more supine position can assist with dislocation of the humeral head
6. The beach chair position may be associated with a slightly higher risk of cerebral hypoperfusion
7. A padded Mayo stand or arm holder can also be useful in providing control and assisting with position of the distal extremity.

G. Incision and dissection:
1. Need adequate exposure to the deep interval

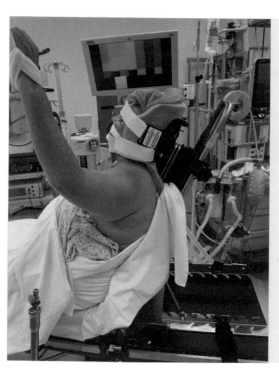

Fig. 3.2 Operating room setup in the beach chair position. Note neutral position of the cervical spine, easy access to the posterior shoulder, and pneumatic arm holder.

2. Skin incision usually placed referencing the coracoid superiorly and the insertion of the pectoralis distally (▶ **Fig. 3.3** and ▶ **Fig. 3.4**)

3. Develop an interval between the medial aspect of the deltoid and the lateral aspect of the pectoralis:

   a. May be easier to identify closer to clavicle

   b. Will usually find the cephalic vein in a fat stripe directly over the interval.

4. Releasing the vein proximally and distally will help mobilize it and prevent tethering at the proximal and distal ends:

   a. The vein may be deep in the interval

   b. Can be absent in cases of prior surgery

   c. In cases of scar or tethering it may be beneficial to move vein medially to prevent iatrogenic laceration from deltoid retraction.

5. Once the interval has been developed, the pectoralis can be elevated off the underlying fascia to further develop the space (▶ **Fig. 3.5**):

   a. This will expose the coracoid and the conjoint tendon coursing distally

   b. The coracoacromial (CA) ligament should also be visualized or palpated

   c. One can also develop the plane between the humeral shaft and the deltoid at the lateral aspect of the humerus at the level of the pectoralis insertion (▶ **Fig. 3.6**).

6. The clavipectoral fascia can be incised lateral to the muscle of the short head of the biceps:

   a. Take care not to plunge to deep to avoid subscapularis injury

   b. Preserve the CA ligament at the top of the release

   c. May release some of the upper border of the pectoralis in tight shoulders.

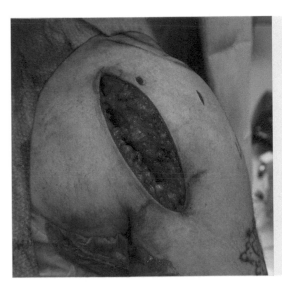

Fig. 3.3 Subcutaneous dissection for the deltopectoral approach.

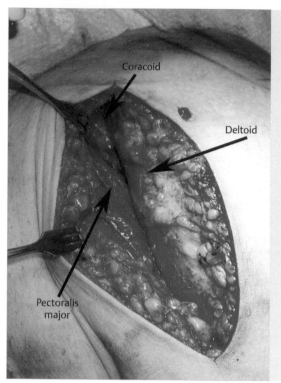

Fig. 3.4 The coracoid is visualized at the superior aspect of the wound. It is easier to distinguish the differing orientation of the pectoralis major and deltoid fibers at this level.

Coracoid

Deltoid

Pectoralis major

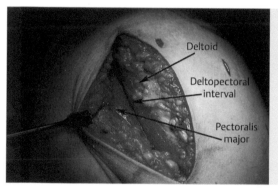

Fig. 3.5 Notice the interval between deltoid and pectoralis major. In this patient, the cephalic vein is deep in the interval and not visible.

Deltoid

Deltopectoral interval

Pectoralis major

7. Once the clavipectoral fascia is incised, the subcoracoid space can be dissected bluntly, exposing the subscapularis:

    a. The axillary nerve can be felt at the inferior aspect of the subscapularis when palpating medially.

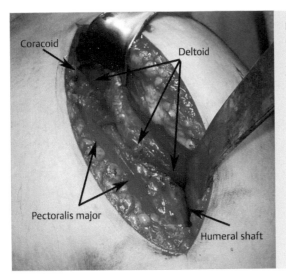

Fig. 3.6 Distal retractor placed around the humeral shaft retracting the deltoid laterally. This exposes the pectoralis insertion. The proximal humerus is still obscured by the overlying deltoid.

8. The subdeltoid space can be developed by dissecting under the CA ligament, but above the rotator cuff

9. Once the subdeltoid space is identified proximally and distally, the remainder of the deltoid can be mobilized off the humeral head and bursa:

    a. The axillary nerve lies on the deep surface of the deltoid, and the surgeon should be careful not to violate the deep fascia of the deltoid

    b. The humeral branch of the posterior circumflex is often at the same level as the axillary nerve and can bleed briskly if not coagulated.

10. The surgeon can use a self-retaining retractor (Kolbel) if desired:

    a. One blade under the conjoined tendon and one blade under the deltoid (▶**Fig. 3.7**)

    b. Excessive retraction can injure the musculocutaneous nerve.

11. In rare cases of severe scarring or poor access, an anteromedial approach reflecting the clavicular origin of the deltoid can be performed. Meticulous reattachment of the deltoid is important to maintain continued functionality

12. If more medial exposure to the plexus or vessels is needed, the surgeon can perform a coracoid osteotomy or conjoint tendon tenotomy.

H. Deep dissection:

    1. A bursectomy can improve visualization

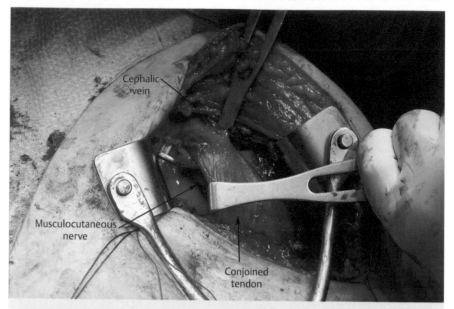

Fig. 3.7 Musculocutaneous nerve seen entering the coracobrachialis when exposing the medial side of the conjoined tendon. This particular patient is undergoing a pectoralis transfer for subscapularis insufficiency.

2. The bicipital groove is usually easily identified and can serve as a landmark during surgical dissection:

a. The long head of the biceps sits in the bicipital groove and can be traced from the upper border of the pectoralis up to the rotator interval

b. As the biceps approaches the interval, it turns medially to enter the joint.

3. The upper rolled border of the subscapularis can usually be palpated in the rotator interval

4. The inferior border of the subscapularis can be identified by the presence of the anterior circumflex artery and its two venae comitantes, often referred to as the "three sisters"

5. Depending on the procedure, different steps can be undertaken at this point

6. Access into the glenohumeral joint can be facilitated through opening the rotator interval or through the subscapularis (▶ **Fig. 3.8**):

a. The rotator interval can be excised to allow better access into joint and identification of structures.

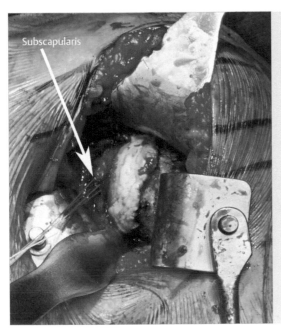

Subscapularis

Fig. 3.8 Proximal humerus exposure for an anatomic total shoulder arthroplasty. One blade of the self-retaining retractor is behind the conjoined tendon, and the other behind the deltoid. A Browne retractor is retracting the deltoid superiorly. A blunt Hohmann is protecting the axillary nerve. The subscapularis has been peeled off the lesser tuberosity and tagged for later repair. Notice the proximal humeral osteophytes.

7. Subscapularis management can be variable (▶ Fig. 3.9):
    a. Lesser tuberosity osteotomy:
        i. A small piece of bone is removed from the lesser tuberosity along with the subscapularis to preserve Sharpey's fibers as well as facilitate direct bony healing when the subscapularis is reattached.
    b. Subscapularis peel:
        i. Elevation of entire subscapularis off the bone starting at the bicipital groove.
    b. Subscapularis split:
        i. Can be used for open Bankart repair, coracoid transfer, or anterior glenoid fracture fixation.
    b. Tenotomy medial to the tuberosity:
        i. Side-to-side tendon repair performed to close.
    e. L-shaped inferior tenotomy.
8. Once the joint is opened, any further capsular releases or intra-articular work can be performed.

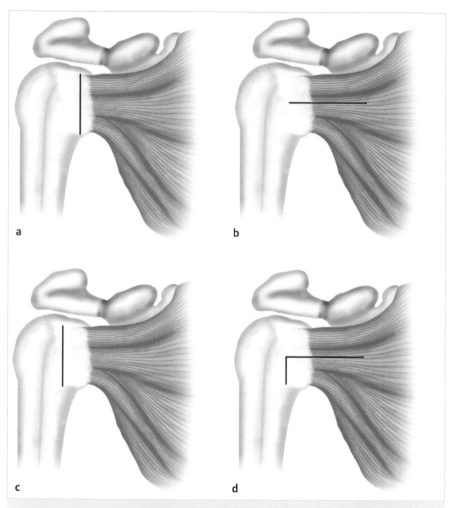

Fig. 3.9 Diagram showing incision lines for subscapularis management. (**a**) Subscapularis tenotomy. (**b**) Subscapularis split. (**c**) Subscapularis peel. (**d**) Inferior subscapularis takedown.

III. Deltoid splitting approach

A. Can be used for rotator cuff repair, proximal humeral fracture fixation, and shoulder arthroplasty

B. Axillary nerve is described as being 5 cm from the lateral edge of the acromion, but it can be closer in smaller patients

C. Incision can be made off the anterolateral corner of the acromion, either in the direction of Langer's lines or the deltoid fibers

D. The acromial attachment of the deltoid can be left intact or reflected off the anterior acromion

E. If distal exposure is needed, the axillary nerve can be palpated and the dissection continued below the nerve. Alternately the nerve can be exposed.

IV. Approach to the acromioclavicular (AC) joint

A. Can be used for resection of the distal clavicle or AC joint reconstruction

B. Any approach to the AC joint should preserve the thick deltotrapezial tissue for closure at the end of the case

C. The skin incision can be in line with the AC joint along Langer's lines or parallel to the clavicle (▶ **Fig. 3.10**)

D. Once skin is divided, full-thickness flaps are elevated off the anterior and posterior surfaces of the AC joint (▶ **Fig. 3.11**)

E. Once the desired procedure is performed, the flaps are repaired to each other or through drill holes.

V. Posterior approaches to the shoulder

A. Can be used in treatment of posterior instability, glenoid osteotomy, oncological surgery, scapular neck fractures, open suprascapular nerve decompression, or posterior fracture dislocations

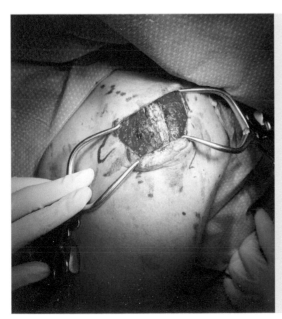

Fig. 3.10 Open approach for reconstruction of an acromioclavicular joint dislocation. The skin incision paralleled Langer's lines and skin flaps were developed to expose medially and laterally. Notice musculoperiosteal flaps elevated in line with clavicle.

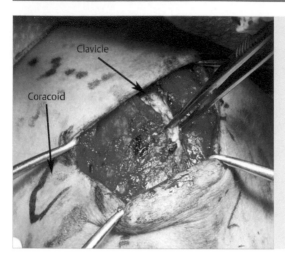

Fig. 3.11 The musculoperiosteal flaps should be full thickness to allow for closure at the end of the procedure.

B. A more extensive Judet approach to the posterior shoulder can be used for scapular body fractures

C. Easiest to position patient in lateral decubitus or prone

D. Skin incision can be along the scapular spine or vertical:

    1. Vertical incision can be made along the soft spot of the joint posteriorly, similar to an arthroscopic portal, or just medial

    2. A laterally placed incision may make access to joint difficult.

E. Once the deltoid is identified it can be split in line with its fibers or elevated off the scapular spine:

    1. The deltoid fibers tend to be oriented in a more horizontal fashion posteriorly.

F. If the deltoid is split, the axillary nerve can be found exiting from the quadrilateral space at the level of the teres minor

G. The deep fascia enveloping the infraspinatus and teres minor can be identified

H. The interval between these two muscles can be developed bluntly toward their insertion on the greater tuberosity

I. Once the two muscles are reflected, the posterior capsule of the joint can be identified and incised as needed

J. For scapular body fractures, a Judet approach can provide extensile exposure:

    1. The incision starts at the spine of the scapula and curves down along the medial edge of the scapular body (▶ **Fig. 3.12**)

    2. The skin and all subcutaneous tissue are elevated as one large flap

    3. The glenohumeral joint and scapular neck can be accessed in a similar method as described above

    4. In addition, this approach will allow plating of the medial border of the scapula.

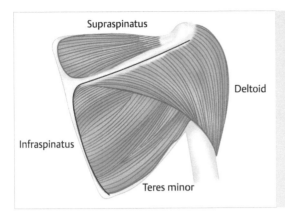

Supraspinatus

Deltoid

Infraspinatus

Teres minor

Fig. 3.12 Line signifying skin incision for posterior Judet approach to the scapula. Once through the subcutaneous tissue, the posterior deltoid can be reflected to reveal the insertion of the teres minor and infraspinatus on the proximal humerus.

Suggested Readings

Chalmers PN, Van Thiel GS, Trenhaile SW. Surgical exposures of the shoulder. J Am Acad Orthop Surg 2016;24(4):250–25810.5435/JAAOS-D-14-00342

Hoppenfeld S; de Boer P, Buckley R. Surgical Exposures in orthopaedics: the anatomic approach. Chapter 1: The Shoulder. Lippincott Williams and Wilkins; 2009

Zlotolow DA, Catalano LW, Barron OA, Glickel SZ. Surgical exposures of the humerus. J Am Acad Orthop Surg 2006;14(13):754–765

4 Shoulder-Spine Syndrome

Scott Wagner and Kelly G. Kilcoyne

Summary

Shoulder and cervical spine patients often have overlapping symptoms, presentations, and complaints. Spine and shoulder surgeons, and all providers seeing patients with cervical and shoulder pathologies, need to be knowledgeable of common shoulder and spine pathologies, presentation, examination, and imaging. Inadequate diagnostic evaluation can and should be avoided utilizing the algorithm proposed in this chapter.

Keywords: Shoulder, cervical, pain, radiculopathy

I. Introduction

A. Shoulder pain:

1. Common complaint; patients may have difficulty localizing exact location of pain and describe more broad upper extremity shoulder and neck pain

2. May result from glenohumeral, acromioclavicular, and/or biceps tendon pathology

3. Can be related to degenerative cervical spine disease and radiculopathy, as roughly a quarter of patients with cervical radiculopathy have symptomatic shoulder impingement:[1]

    a. May also be referred to as cervical facetogenic pain.[2,3]

4. Often difficult to differentiate referred cervical radiculopathy from glenohumeral or subacromial shoulder pain secondary to complexity of pain patterns and interactions between joint articulations[4]

5. In addition, there may be an association between spinal kyphosis and scapular impingement syndrome,[5] and increased thoracic kyphosis and spinal inclination angles have been shown to be risk factors for limitations in active shoulder motion[6] and development of scapular dyskinesis:

    a. It is not known how many shoulder surgeries are performed for mis or undiagnosed cervical pathology as a result of inadequate evaluation and workup of cervical spine pathology as possible primary pain generator

    b. It is not known how cervical and shoulder surgeries may affect shoulder alignment and mechanics

    c. There is no standard algorithm for clinicians, shoulder and spine specialists specifically, to evaluate and differentiate overlapping causes and presentations of "shoulder pain."

6. The interaction between the cervical spine and the shoulder is similar to those described in Hip Spine Syndrome.[7,8] The goal of this review chapter is to review the basic approach to the shoulder-spine patient including an algorithm for the evaluation and diagnostic workup for the complaint of "shoulder pain."

II. Diagnosis

A. History:

1. Common sources of shoulder pain (▶ **Fig 4.1a, b**):

   a. Often increased pain with arm abduction[9]

   b. Pain over acromioclavicular joint (ACJ) and adjacent to lateral acromion

   c. Rotator cuff tears (RTC):

      i. Increased incidence of both symptomatic and asymptomatic tears with age

      ii. Numbness and tingling past the elbow, even into palm, can be seen in patients with RTC tears/tendonitis and subacromial bursitis. Pain that extends into the finger tips is more commonly from cervical pathology.

   d. Biceps/superior labral anterior to posterior (SLAP), anterior and deep shoulder pain

   e. Glenohumeral osteoarthritis (OA)—global pain, typically increased with movement

   f. Shoulder instability

   g. Scapular dyskinesis/trapezial pain—typically posterior and periscapular pain.

2. Common cervical radiculopathy complaints:

   a. Often pain relief with arm abduction[9]

   b. Numbness/tingling in arm, forearm, and hand

   c. Review of dermatomes/myotomes, exiting nerve root anatomy:

      i. C4: Base of neck/upper shoulder

      ii. C5: Shoulder/deltoid, lateral arm

      iii. C6: Shoulder, lateral arm, radial forearm, thumb/IF.

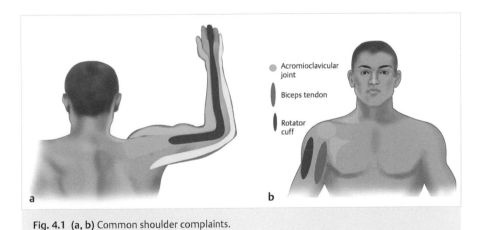

Acromioclavicular joint

Biceps tendon

Rotator cuff

a

b

Fig. 4.1 (a, b) Common shoulder complaints.

B. Physical examination:

   1. Shoulder:

      a. Impingement tests—Neer/Hawkins, cross-arm test, and ACJ tenderness to palpation

      b. Biceps/SLAP—Speed/Yergason's test, O'brien's test, dynamic load and shear

      c. RTC—Strength testing, Jobe's test, empty can test:

         i. Drop arm, painful arc.

      d. Instability:

         i. Anterior and posterior translation

         ii. Apprehension, Jerk test.

      e. Range of motion.

   2. Cervical spine:

      a. Paraspinal/trapezius tenderness and pain

      b. Motor examination

      c. Spurling's sign: High specificity for radiculopathy, but only 30–50% sensitivity and often performed incorrectly.[10,11]

      d. Squeeze arm test: First described in 2013, the test involves compression of the upper third of the symptomatic arm, ACJ, and anterolateral-subacromial area:[12]

         i. The test is considered positive if visual analog scale (VAS) pain level reached or exceeded 3/10

         ii. As described, the test has a sensitivity of 96% and specificity ranging from 91 to 100% for cervical nerve root pathology.

III. Diagnostic tests

A. Plain radiography:

   1. Shoulder:

      a. Indicated in patients whose physical examination findings suggest the shoulder as the primary source[4]

      b. Anteroposterior (AP), Grashey AP, scapular "Y," and axial views.

   2. Cervical spine:

      a. AP, lateral, and flexion/extension:

         i. Osteophytosis, disk collapse, static or dynamic spondylolisthesis

         ii. Indicated in patients with shoulder complaints who also complain of axial neck pain, and/or radicular symptoms or who have peripheral weakness in strength testing.

B. Advanced imaging:

   1. Shoulder:

      a. Magnetic resonance imaging (MRI) to evaluate for RTC tears, labral tears, biceps abnormality, cartilage injury, and/or arthritic joint changes.

   2. Cervical:
      a. MRI:
         i. Evaluate for central versus foraminal stenosis, myelomalacia, and perineural or facet cysts
         ii. Computed tomography (CT) myelogram if unable to obtain MRI.
C. Diagnostic/therapeutic injections:
   1. Shoulder: Only in rare instances are injections performed prior to obtaining an MRI as this can potentially guide treatment:
      a. Subacromial injections: In patients with impingement findings or evidence of subacromial bursitis or partial RTC tears
      b. Glenohumeral injections: To address any potential intra-articular sources of pain including biceps, labrum, and RTC
      c. ACJ injections: Can be done in isolation in patients with isolated ACJ symptoms.
   2. Cervical:
      a. Selective nerve root block (SNRB), interlaminar epidural steroid injection:
         i. Dangers associated with injections in C-spine
         ii. Cervical SNRB pain relief may correlate with symptom relief after surgical intervention, but patients experiencing no effect after injection still may have pain relief with surgery:[13]
            • Questionable diagnostic utility.
D. Electrodiagnostics:
   1. Used if diagnosis remains unclear but cervical is suspected to be the main etiology[4]
   2. Often negative in purely sensory radiculopathy.

IV. Differential diagnosis

A. Also consider: Peripheral vascular disease, diabetic neuropathy, and acute cardiac pathology
B. Neuralgic amyotrophy (Parsonage-Turner syndrome)
C. Uncommon shoulder conditions: avascular necrosis, metastases, fractures, and cysts
D. Thoracic outlet syndrome:
   1. Cervical ribs (▶ Fig. 4.2).

V. Management

A. Surgical management is only considered after a trial of conservative measures, regardless of the etiology, in the absence of progressive neurologic deficits. In patients with concurrent pathology, the predominant complaint should guide treatment.

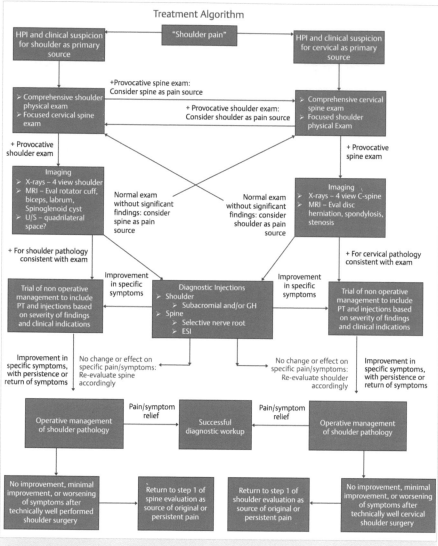

Fig. 4.2 Treatment algorithm.

1. Shoulder:
   a. RTC repair in symptomatic patients with full- or nearly full-thickness tear
   b. Shoulder arthroscopy with biceps tenodesis in patients with degeneration or tearing of superior labrum/biceps complex
   c. Labral repair in patients with recurrent glenohumeral instability.
2. Cervical:
   a. Anterior cervical discectomy and fusion (ACDF)/cervical disk arthroplasty (CDA)
   b. Keyhole foraminotomy.

References

1. Date ES, Gray LA. Electrodiagnostic evidence for cervical radiculopathy and suprascapular neuropathy in shoulder pain. Electromyogr Clin Neurophysiol 1996;36(6):333–339
2. Dwyer A, Aprill C, Bogduk N. Cervical zygapophyseal joint pain patterns. I: A study in normal volunteers. Spine 1990;15(6)) ::453–457
3. Gerber C, Galantay RV, Hersche O. The pattern of pain produced by irritation of the acromioclavicular joint and the subacromial space. J Shoulder Elbow Surg 1998;7(4):352–355
4. Bokshan SL, DePasse JM, Eltorai AE, Paxton ES, Green A, Daniels AH. An evidence-based approach to differentiating the cause of shoulder and cervical spine pain. Am J Med 2016;129(9):913–918
5. Otoshi K, Takegami M, Sekiguchi M, et al. Association between kyphosis and subacromial impingement syndrome: LOHAS study. J Shoulder Elbow Surg 2014;23(12):e300–e307
6. Imagama S, Hasegawa Y, Wakao N, Hirano K, Muramoto A, Ishiguro N. Impact of spinal alignment and back muscle strength on shoulder range of motion in middle-aged and elderly people in a prospective cohort study. Eur Spine J 2014;23(7):1414–1419
7. Offierski CM, MacNab I. Hip-spine syndrome. Spine 1983;8(3):316–321
8. Devin CJ, McCullough KA, Morris BJ, Yates AJ, Kang JD. Hip-spine syndrome. J Am Acad Orthop Surg 2012;20(7):434–442
9. Mitchell C, Adebajo A, Hay E, Carr A. Shoulder pain: diagnosis and management in primary care. BMJ 2005;331(7525):1124–1128
10. Tong HC, Haig AJ, Yamakawa K. The Spurling test and cervical radiculopathy. Spine 2002;27(2):156–159
11. Wainner RS, Fritz JM, Irrgang JJ, Boninger ML, Delitto A, Allison S. Reliability and diagnostic accuracy of the clinical examination and patient self-report measures for cervical radiculopathy. Spine 2003;28(1):52–62
12. Gumina S, Carbone S, Albino P, Gurzi M, Postacchini F. Arm squeeze test: a new clinical test to distinguish neck from shoulder pain. Eur Spine J 2013;22(7):1558–1563
13. Antoniadis A, Dietrich TJ, Farshad M. Does pain relief by CT-guided indirect cervical nerve root injection with local anesthetics and steroids predict pain relief after decompression surgery for cervical nerve root compression? Acta Neurochir (Wien) 2016;158(10):1869–1874

5 Shoulder Imaging

Joseph Ferraro and Matthew Binkley

Summary

Along with thorough history and physical exam, appropriate imaging is integral to accurate diagnosis and treatment of shoulder pathology. Understanding the various shoulder imaging options can help confirm diagnosis while minimizing unnecessary testing. In this chapter, many imaging choices will be discussed, paired with corresponding pathology to add to your clinical armamentarium.

Keywords: Radiography, X-ray, MRI, CT, MR arthrogram

I. Radiography

A. The initial imaging modality for evaluation of the shoulder

B. Provides little information on soft tissue around the shoulder

C. Shoulder series should consist of at least two orthogonal views

D. Trauma evaluation includes:

    1. True anteroposterior aka Grashey (▶**Fig. 5.1**):

        a. Erect, sitting, or supine with patient rotated 30–45 degrees in relation to the image detector

        b. Evaluate glenohumeral joint, fracture (proximal humerus, clavicle, scapula, and ribs), and proximal humeral migration.

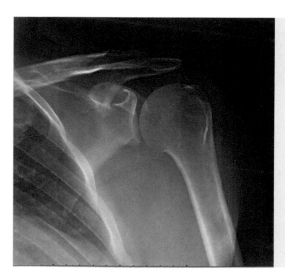

Fig. 5.1 Grashey.

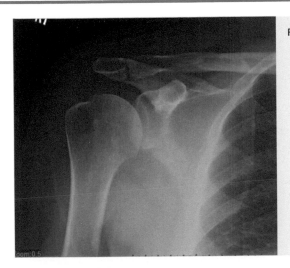

Fig. 5.2 Anteroposterior (AP).

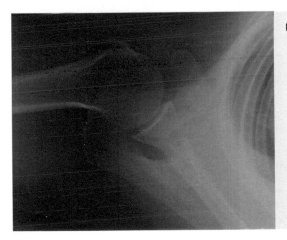

Fig. 5.3 Axillary lateral.

2. Anteroposterior (AP) (▶Fig. 5.2):
   a. Erect, sitting, or supine with beam perpendicular to body
   b. Allows for viewing of shoulder in anatomical position
   c. Utility similar to Grashey view with poorer view of glenohumeral joint.
3. Axillary lateral (▶Fig. 5.3):
   a. Supine, arm abducted with beam parallel to body
   b. Evaluate joint congruency, direction of dislocation, and glenoid pathology
   c. Velpeau view can be used for patient who cannot abduct the arm:
      i. Patient erect leaning backwards over cassette.

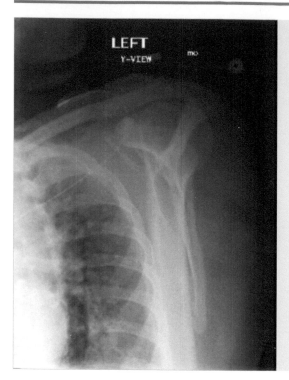

Fig. 5.4 Scapular Y lateral.

4. Scapular Y lateral (▶**Fig. 5.4**):
    a. Sitting or erect, anterior oblique view with scapula in profile
    b. Evaluate acromion type scapular fracture.
E. Additional views:
    1. AP in external or internal rotation (▶**Fig. 5.5a, b**):
        a. Same positioning as AP with humerus externally or internally rotated
        b. External rotation:
            i. Greater tuberosity on profile.
        c. Internal rotation:
            i. Lesser tuberosity on profile, best view of Hill-Sachs lesion.
    2. Stryker notch (▶**Fig. 5.6**):
        a. Arm extended over head with elbow flexed; beam directed at mid axilla with 10 degrees caudal tilt
        b. Excellent visibility of posterolateral humeral head for Hill-Sachs lesion.

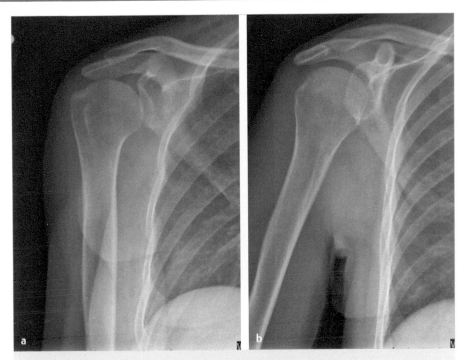

Fig. 5.5 (a, b) Anteroposterior (AP) in external or internal rotation.

3. Supraspinatus outlet aka Neer (▶**Fig. 5.7**):
   a. Affected shoulder on X-ray plate while rotating the other shoulder out 40 degrees; PA view with beam at 10 degrees caudal tilt
   b. Ideal view for evaluating acromion type as well as supraspinatus impingement.
4. West point axillary:
   a. Patient prone with arm abducted 90 degrees and forearm off table. Beam aimed at mid axilla, 25 degrees from midline and 25 degrees caudal tilt
   b. Provides better view of anteroinferior glenoid for evaluation of bony Bankart lesion.
5. Apical oblique aka Garth:
   a. Patient erect or sitting with back against receiver and affected side's hand resting on unaffected side's shoulder. Beam at 30–45 degrees in coronal plane and 45 degrees caudal tilt

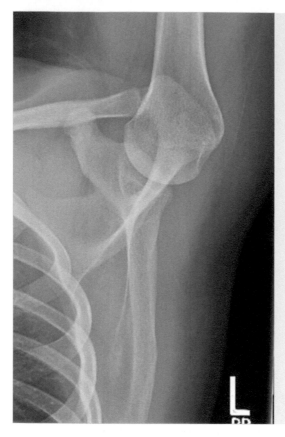

Fig. 5.6 Stryker notch.

    b.   Provides improved view of glenohumeral joint to evaluate for Bankart and Hill-Sachs lesions

    c.   Can be used in place of axillary or scapular Y to evaluate for glenohumeral dislocation.

6.   Serendipity/Hobbs (▶ **Fig. 5.8**):

    a.   Serendipity = Patient supine with beam 40 degrees tilt from horizontal

    b.   Hobbs = Patient bent over cassette with arms forward flexed and head resting in hands

    c.   Evaluate for sternoclavicular dislocation.

7.   Zanca (▶ **Fig. 5.9**):

    a.   Patient erect or sitting with back against cassette; beam aimed at shoulder with 10–15 degrees cephalic tilt

    b.   Evaluate acromioclavicular joint en face for separation or arthritis.

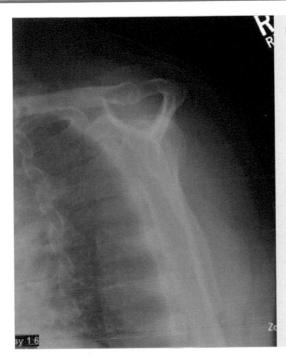

Fig. 5.7 Neer.

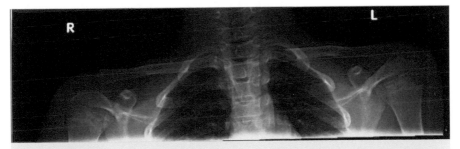

Fig. 5.8 Serendipity.

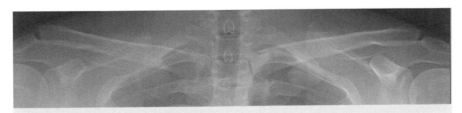

Fig. 5.9 Zanca.

II. Computed tomography

A. Better bony detail compared to radiography and magnetic resonance imaging (MRI) with higher radiation load

B. Superior soft tissue detail compared to radiography especially with addition of contrast although still inferior to MRI

C. Images reformatted in multiple planes to provide details useful in total shoulder arthroplasty, trauma, and oncological surgical planning:

    1. Axial (►Fig. 5.10):

        a. Useful for visualization of fractures, degenerative disease, glenoid morphology, dislocation, and bony defects (Hill-Sachs, reverse Hill-Sachs, Bankart).

    2. Sagittal (►Fig. 5.11):

        a. Useful for visualization of fractures, glenoid morphology, and calcific tendonosis.

    3. Coronal (►Fig. 5.12):

        a. Useful for visualization of fractures, arthritis, and proximal humeral migration.

D. Three-dimensional reconstruction (►Fig. 5.13):

    1. Useful for visualization of glenoid version for total shoulder arthroplasty surgical planning as well as better visualization of complex fracture patterns of the scapula.

E. Computed tomography (CT) arthrography (►Fig. 5.14):

    1. Injection of iodinated contrast dye into joint

    2. Allows for better visualization of joint space and evaluation of rotator cuff and labral integrity

    3. Commonly used when patient has had prior surgery or shoulder arthroplasty procedure, or there are concerns for labral pathology.

III. Magnetic resonance imaging

A. Best imaging modality for evaluating soft tissues as well as bony contusion

B. T1 weighted (►Fig. 5.15):

    1. Hyperintense = Fat

    2. Hypointense = Fluid, bones, tendons, ligaments, muscles

    3. Generally considered to be best for viewing anatomy

    4. Useful for visualization of bony Bankart and Hill-Sachs lesions.

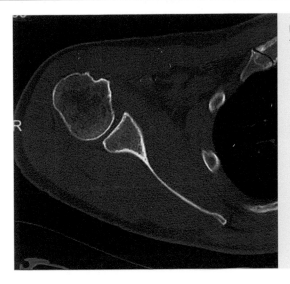

Fig. 5.10 Computed tomography (CT), axial.

C. T2 weighted (▶ **Fig. 5.16**):
    1. Hyperintense = Fluid, bone marrow.
D. Hypointense = Bones, ligaments, muscles
    1. Generally considered to be best for viewing pathology
    2. Useful for visualizing rotator cuff tears (especially subscapularis tendon), hairline fracture, and contusion.
E. Short tau inversion recovery (STIR) (▶ **Fig. 5.17**):
    1. Fat suppressed and fluid/edema accentuated
    2. Useful in evaluating edema versus fatty infiltration in rotator cuff tears.
F. MR arthrogram (▶ **Fig. 5.18**):
    1. Gadolinium contrast installed into joint
    2. Excellent visibility of superior labral anterior to posterior (SLAP), glenolabral articular disruption (GLAD), humeral avulsion of the glenohumeral ligament (HAGL), and anterior labroligamentous periosteal sleeve avulsion (ALPSA) lesions
    3. Superior soft tissue visualization compared to CT arthrogram.

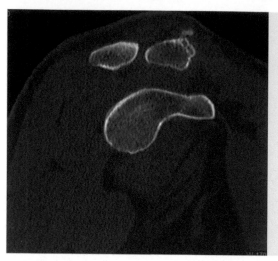

Fig. 5.11 Computed tomography (CT), sagittal.

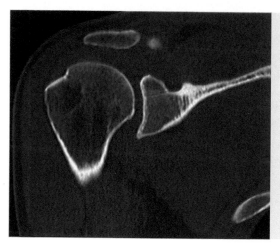

Fig. 5.12 Computed tomography (CT), coronal.

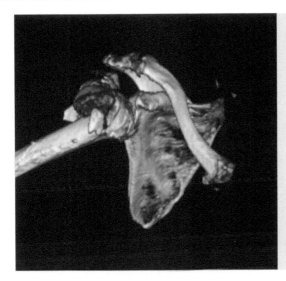

Fig. 5.13 Three-dimensional reconstruction.

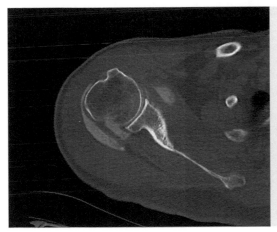

Fig. 5.14 Computed tomography (CT) arthrogram.

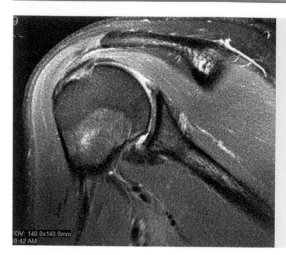

Fig. 5.15 T1 magnetic resonance imaging (MRI).

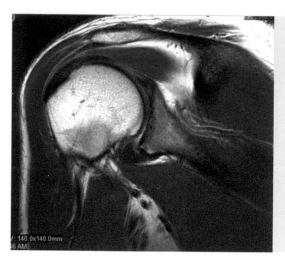

Fig. 5.16 T2 magnetic resonance imaging (MRI).

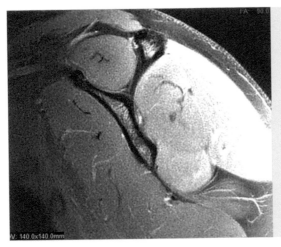

Fig. 5.17 Short tau inversion recovery (STIR) magnetic resonance imaging (MRI).

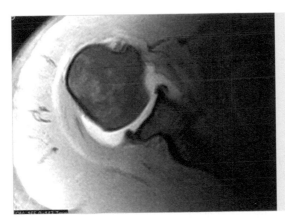

Fig. 5.18 Magnetic resonance imaging (MRI) arthrogram.

Suggested Readings

Goud A, Segal D, Hedayati P, Pan JJ, Weissman BN. Radiographic evaluation of the shoulder. Eur J Radiol 2008;68(1):2–15

Iannotti JP, Zlatkin MB, Esterhai JL, Kressel HY, Dalinka MK, Spindler KP. Magnetic resonance imaging of the shoulder: sensitivity, specificity, and predictive value. J Bone Joint Surg Am 1991;73(1):17–29

Jensen KL, Tirman P. Radiographic evaluation of shoulder problems. In: Matsen FA, Lippitt SB. Rockwood and Matsen's The Shoulder. 5th ed. Elsevier; 2017:135–168:135–168

Lecouvet FE, Simoni P, Koutaïssoff S, Vande Berg BC, Malghem J, Dubuc JE. Multidetector spiral CT arthrography of the shoulder: clinical applications and limits, with MR arthrography and arthroscopic correlations. Eur J Radiol 2008;68(1):120–136

Murphy A, Gilcrease-Garcia B. "Shoulder Series | Radiology Reference Article." Radiopaedia.org, radiopaedia. org/articles/shoulder-series Murphy A, Gilcrease-Garcia B. "Shoulder Series | Radiology Reference Article." Radiopaedia.org, radiopaedia.org/articles/shoulder-series

Sanders TG, Jersey SL. Conventional radiography of the shoulder. Semin Roentgenol 2005;40(3):207–222

6 Ultrasound of the Shoulder

Paul S. Ragusa and Uma Srikumaran

Summary

Shoulder ultrasound is a safe, efficient, and cost-effective method used to dynamically evaluate the rotator cuff tendons, biceps tendon, and other structures of the shoulder joint. It is accurate for detecting large and massive rotator cuff tears and is comparable to magnetic resonance imaging (MRI) in both sensitivity and specificity.

Keywords: Shoulder, ultrasonography, rotator cuff, efficiency, diagnosis

I. General principles

A. Ultrasound basics:[1]
    1. Ultrasound uses the principles of sonar developed for ships at sea
    2. A transducer is used to produce sound waves
    3. When the sound waves encounter a border between two tissues that conduct sound differently some of the sound waves bounce back creating an echo
    4. The transducer detects the returning echoes which are analyzed by a computer and transformed into an image
    5. The more dense the tissue, the brighter the appearance on the image.

B. Definitions:[1]
    1. Echogenicity:
        a. The type of echo display: Anechoic/hypoechoic/hyperechoic.
    2. Anechoic:
        a. Without echoes; black; fluid filled structures; in shoulder pathology, anechoic signals typically represents pathology (e.g., effusion, tissue tear).
    3. Hypoechoic:
        a. With low-level echoes; grays; more solid structure.
    4. Hyperechoic:
        a. Bright echoes; white; dense or strong reflector.
    5. Isoechoic:
        a. Same echogenicity.
    6. Attenuation:
        a. Loss of energy as a sound pulse travels through a medium.
    7. Long-axis:
        a. Along the length of the structure.

8. Short-axis:
    a. Across the width of the structure.
9. Anisotropy:
    a. An artifactual hypoechoic appearance of a normal hyperechoic structure that occurs because the transducer is not perpendicular to the structure being imaged
    b. You can help combat this by maintaining an angle of close to 90 degrees between the probe and the structure of interest.
10. Frequency:
    a. The range of sound waves produced by a transducer (measured in MHz)
    b. The higher the frequency the better image detail, but lesser the penetration; a high-frequency transducer (12 to 15 MHz) is typically used to evaluate the shoulder
    c. The lower the frequency the lesser image detail, but better the penetration; lower frequency transducer (9 MHz) may be used to achieve greater tissue penetration, which may be necessary when evaluating deeper structures such as when evaluating patients with a large body habitus.

C. Advantages of ultrasound:
1. Cost-effective
2. Safe
3. Improves efficiency in the management of rotator cuff disease[2]
4. Dynamic
5. Accurate for detecting large and massive rotator cuff tears[3,6]
6. Comparable to magnetic resonance imaging (MRI) in both sensitivity and specificity[7]
7. Can be used in patients with contraindications to MRI (pacemaker, claustrophobia, etc.)
8. Accurate for evaluating the rotator cuff in shoulders that have undergone an operation:
    a. Less susceptibility to suture anchor artifact.[8]
9. Allows for image guided injections.

D. Disadvantages:
1. Long learning curve:
    a. 100 ultrasound examinations recommended prior to clinical application.[9,10]
2. Operator dependent
3. Difficult with obese/well-muscled patients
4. Less sensitive for detecting partial-thickness rotator cuff tears and ruptures of the biceps[6]
5. Does not evaluate intraarticular structures well (labrum, biceps anchor, etc.).

II. Normal shoulder examination

A. Long head biceps tendon (LHBT):

    1. Patient position:

        a. Performed with shoulder in neutral or slight internal rotation, elbow flexed 90 degrees, and forearm supinated and resting on the patient's lap.

    2. Short-axis image (▶ **Fig. 6.1a, b**):

        a. Hold the probe transversely with respect to the longitudinal axis of the LHBT

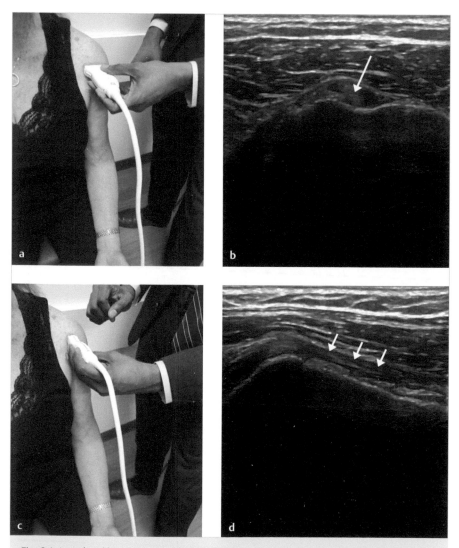

Fig. 6.1 Long head biceps tendon (LHBT). (**a**) Patient and probe position for imaging the LHBT in short-axis. (**b**) Short-axis image of LHBT (*arrow*). (**c**) Patient and probe position for imaging the LHBT in long-axis. (**d**) Long-axis image of LHBT (*short arrows*).

    b. Image is equivalent to an axial view on MRI

    c. Normal appearance:

        i. Homogeneous, round, or ovoid hyperechoic structure (2–4 mm thick) located in the bicipital groove with trace amount of fluid within its tendon sheath.

3. Long-axis image (▶ **Fig. 6.1c, d**):

    a. Rotate the probe 90 degrees so that it is oriented along the longitudinal axis of the LHBT

    b. Image is equivalent to a sagittal-oblique view on MRI

    c. This image is typically used when performing a biceps tendon sheath injection

    d. Normal appearance:

        i. Smooth and fibrillar.

B. Subscapularis tendon:

1. Patient position:

    a. Performed with shoulder in external rotation, elbow flexed 90 degrees, and forearm supinated

    b. External rotation delivers the tendon out from underneath the coracoid process.

2. Long-axis image (▶ **Fig. 6.2a, b**):

    a. Hold the probe so that it is aligned along the longitudinal axis of the subscapularis muscle fibers

    b. Image is equivalent to an axial view on MRI

    c. Normal appearance:

        i. Tendon is hyperechoic and convex shaped, tapering toward its insertion on the lesser tuberosity. Normal hypoechoic muscle should not be mistaken for fluid.

3. Short-axis image (▶ **Fig. 6.2c, d**):

    a. Rotate the probe 90 degrees so that it is oriented perpendicular to the subscapularis muscle fibers

    b. Image is equivalent to a sagittal-oblique view on MRI

    c. Good for evaluating superior subscapularis tendon tears.

C. Supraspinatus tendon:

1. Patient position:

    a. Patient is directed to place the palm of his or her hand on the ipsilateral hip or buttock, with elbow flexed and adducted against the body

    b. This allows the supraspinatus tendon to come out from underneath the acromion process.

2. Long-axis image (▶ **Fig. 6.3a, b**):

    a. Hold the probe so that it is aligned along the longitudinal axis of the supraspinatus muscle fibers. The muscle fibers and tendon of the supraspinatus are oriented anterolaterally

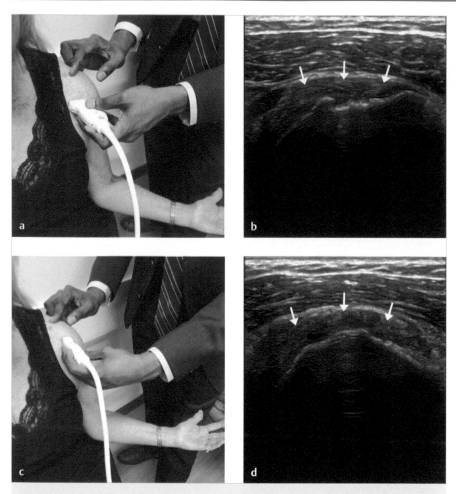

Fig. 6.2 Subscapularis tendon. (**a**) Patient and probe position for imaging the subscapularis in long-axis. (**b**) Long-axis image of subscapularis tendon (*arrows*). (**c**) Patient and probe position for imaging the subscapularis in short-axis. (**d**) Short-axis image of subscapularis tendon (*arrows*).

b. While maintaining probe in the same axis, scan from anterior to posterior

c. Image is equivalent to a coronal-oblique view on MRI

d. Biceps tendon marks the anterior leading edge of the supraspinatus. Posterior supraspinatus is marked by the change in shape of the greater tuberosity, from ledge-like to flat. This area of transition is where the fibers of the posterior supraspinatus and anterior infraspinatus interdigitate and may be mistaken for a tear if the orientation of the probe is not corrected.

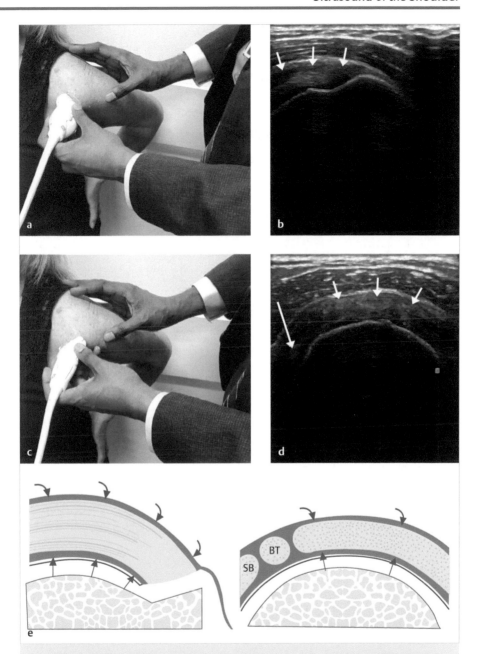

Fig. 6.3 Supraspinatus tendon. (a) Patient and probe position for imaging the supraspinatus in long-axis. (b) Long-axis image of the supraspinatus tendon (*arrows*). (c) Patient and probe position for imaging the supraspinatus in short-axis. Note long head biceps tendon (LHBT) visualized anterior to the supraspinatus tendon (*arrow*). (d) Short-axis image of the supraspinatus tendon (*short arrows*). (e) Illustration of supraspinatus in long-axis (left) and short axis (right) showing the articular (*arrows*) and bursal (*curved arrows*) surfaces of the supraspinatus tendon. BT, biceps tendon; ST, supraspinatus tendon. (Adapted from Jacobson JA. Fundamentals of Musculoskeletal Ultrasound.)

  e. Normal appearance:

    i. Smooth, hyperechoic, and fibrillar, tapering at its insertion or footprint.

  f. Subacromial-subdeltoid bursa:

    i. The subacromial-subdeltoid bursa is located between the rotator cuff and the overlying deltoid muscle and acromion

    ii. The bursae is a potential space which consists of a thin hypoechoic band measuring less than 2 mm surrounded by a thin hyperechoic line superficial and deep to this. It should have a smooth appearance throughout.

 3. Short-axis image (▶ **Fig. 6.4c d**):

  a. Turn probe 90 degrees so that it is aligned perpendicular to the longitudinal axis of the supraspinatus muscle fibers

  b. Image is equivalent to a sagittal-oblique view on MRI

  c. While maintaining probe in the same axis, scan from medial to lateral

  d. Normal appearance:

    i. The hyperechoic lines of the humeral head and the bursal border of the supraspinatus parallel each other.

D. Infraspinatus tendon:

 1. Patient position:

  a. Performed with shoulder in neutral rotation, elbow flexed 90 degrees, and forearm supinated and resting on the patient's lap.

 2. Long-axis image (▶ **Fig. 6.4a, b**):

  a. Hold the probe below the scapular spine. Align it so that it is along the longitudinal axis of the infraspinatus muscle fibers

  b. Image is equivalent to an axial view on MRI

  c. Normal appearance:

    i. Similar fibrillar pattern as supraspinatus tendon; tendon is hyperechoic and tapers toward its insertion on the greater tuberosity. Central tendon can be identified within the surrounding hypoechoic infraspinatus muscle.

 3. Short-axis image (▶ **Fig. 6.4c, d**):

  a. Turn probe 90 degrees so that it is aligned perpendicular to the longitudinal axis of the infraspinatus muscle fibers

  b. Image appears similar to sagittal-oblique MRI

  c. While maintaining probe in the same axis, scan from medial to lateral

  d. Normal appearance:

    i. Similar echogenicity as supraspinatus.

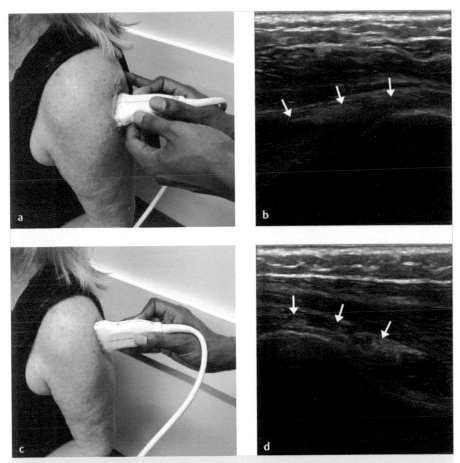

Fig. 6.4 Infraspinatus tendon. **(a)** Patient and probe position for imaging the infraspinatus in long-axis. **(b)** Long-axis image of infraspinatus tendon (*arrows*). **(c)** Patient and probe position for imaging the infraspinatus in short-axis. **(d)** Short-axis image of infraspinatus tendon (*arrows*).

E. Coracoid and anterior glenohumeral joint:

1. Patient position:

   a. Performed with shoulder in external rotation, elbow flexed 90 degrees, and forearm supinated.

2. Long-axis image (▶ Fig. 6.5a, b):

   a. Hold the probe in the same position as the long-axis image for the subscapularis tendon (i.e., along the longitudinal axis of the subscapularis muscle fibers). While maintaining the probe in this axis, slide the probe medially

   b. Image is equivalent to an axial view on MRI

61

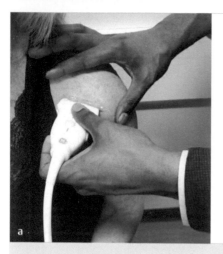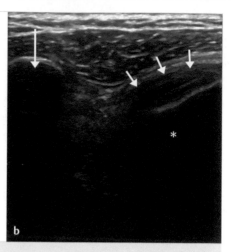

Fig. 6.5 Coracoid and anterior glenohumeral joint. (a) Patient and probe position for long-axis view of coracoid and anterior glenohumeral joint. (b) Long-axis image of coracoid (*arrow*), subscapularis (*short arrows*) and humeral head (*asterisk*).

    c. Typically used for measuring the coracohumeral interval and performing anterior glenohumeral joint injections

    d. Normal appearance:

        i. There should be an absence of fluid inside the joint.

F. Posterior glenohumeral joint:

  1. Patient position:

    a. Performed with shoulder in neutral rotation, elbow flexed 90 degrees, and forearm supinated and resting on the patient's lap.

  2. Long-axis image (▶**Fig. 6.6a–c**):

    a. Hold the probe in the same position as the long-axis image for the infraspinatus (i.e., along the longitudinal axis of the infraspinatus muscle fibers). While maintaining the probe in this axis, slide medially

    b. Image is equivalent to an axial view on MRI

    c. Typically used for posterior glenohumeral joint injections for conditions such as adhesive capsulitis or degenerative joint disease

    d. Normal appearance:

        i. There should be an absence of any fluid inside the joint.

G. Acromioclavicular (AC) joint:

  1. Patient position:

    a. Performed with shoulder in neutral rotation, elbow flexed 90 degrees, and forearm resting on the patient's lap.

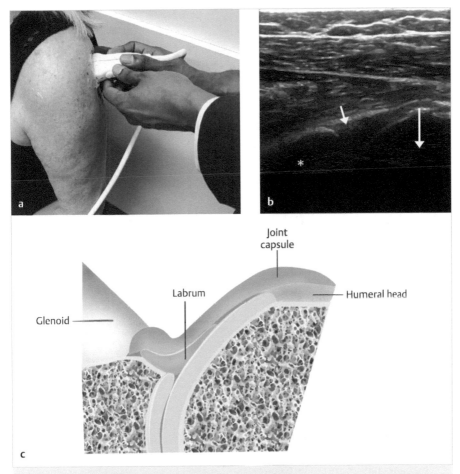

Fig. 6.6 Posterior glenohumeral joint. **(a)** Patient and probe position for long-axis view of the posterior glenohumeral joint. **(b)** Long-axis image of the posterior glenohumeral joint showing the humeral head (*long arrow*) and glenoid (*asterisk*) and labrum (*short arrow*). **(c)** Illustration of posterior glenohumeral joint.

2. Long-axis image (▶ **Fig. 6.7a, b**):

    a. Hold the probe so that it is aligned along the longitudinal axis of the distal end of the clavicle

    b. Image is equivalent to a coronal view

    c. Used for AC joint injections

    d. Normal appearance:

        i. There should be no abnormal joint widening or narrowing, joint margin irregularity, step-off, or capsular bulging.

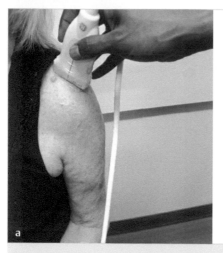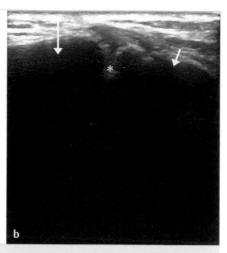

Fig. 6.7 Acromioclavicular(AC) joint. (a) Patient and probe position for long-axis view of the AC joint. (b) Long-axis image of the AC joint (*asterisk*), distal clavicle (*long arrow*), acromion (*short arrow*).

III. Pathologic conditions

A.   LHBT:

    1.   Long head biceps tendinosis:

        a.   Thickening, loss of normal echogenicity, and loss of normal fibrillar pattern.

    2.   Partial-thickness (longitudinal intrasubstance) tear:

        a.   May occur due to chronic tendinosis

        b.   Results in an anechoic void within the tendon, without complete discontinuity

        c.   These tears are often longitudinally oriented.

    3.   Full-thickness tear:

        a.   Complete tear with distal retraction is characterized by nonvisualization of the tendon within the intertubercular groove (i.e., "empty groove")

        b.   Echogenic material may be present in the groove

        c.   Clinically correlate with a Popeye deformity

        d.   If an empty groove is visualized, assess for medial dislocation of the tendon which may signify a tear of the subscapularis tendon.

B. Subscapularis tendon:

   1. Subcoracoid impingement:

      a. Dynamic scanning can be used to confirm impingement between the coracoid and the underlying subscapularis tendon by internally and externally rotating the shoulder.

   2. Full-thickness tear:

      a. Medial subluxation of the LHBT deep to the subscapularis tendon and into the glenohumeral joint signifies a full-thickness tear of the subscapularis tendon.

C. Supraspinatus and infraspinatus:

   1. Rotator cuff tendinosis:

      a. Tendon appears heterogeneous or hypoechoic, with tendon thickening, and loss of the normal fibrillar pattern.

   2. Partial-thickness rotator cuff tears (▶ Fig. 6.8a–f):

      a. Focal area of hypoechogenicity or mixed echogenicity involving one side of the tendon, but not extending through the entire thickness

      b. May be bursal-sided, articular-side, or intrasubstance.

   3. Full-thickness rotator cuff tears (▶ Fig. 6.8g, h):

      a. Ultrasound is a reliable method for diagnosis of full-thickness rotator cuff tears, with sensitivity and specificity over 90%

      b. Ultrasound is less reliable to pick up partial-thickness tears

      c. Full-thickness tears are visualized as a hypoechoic or anechoic gap within the rotator cuff

      d. When looking at the sagittal view, the hyperechoic lines of the bursal border and articular head are parallel to each other; in the case of a rotator cuff, the bursal border may have a concave contour as the deltoid drops into the cuff defect

      e. Alternatively, a greatly retracted tear can result in nonvisualization of the rotator cuff tendon

      f. Dynamic contraction test: Ask the patient to abduct his or her shoulder against resistance. This isometric contraction is used to uncover nondisplaced full-thickness tears, or significant partial-thickness tears.

   4. Subacromial-subdeltoid bursa:

      a. Abnormalities of the bursa manifest with increased fluid within and distention of the bursa, and/or by bursal wall thickening.

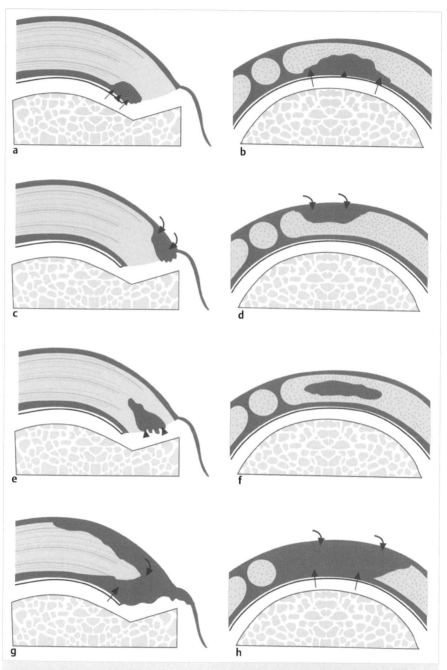

Fig. 6.8 Pathologic conditions of the supraspinatus tendon. (**a**) Long-axis and (**b**) short-axis of articular-sided partial-thickness rotator cuff tear. (**c**) Long-axis and (**d**) short-axis of bursal-sided partial-thickness rotator cuff tear. (**e**) Long-axis and (**f**) short-axis illustration of interstitial partial-thickness rotator cuff tear. (**g**) Long-axis and (**h**) short-axis illustration of full-thickness rotator cuff tear. (Adapted from Jacobson JA. Fundamentals of Musculoskeletal Ultrasound.)

References

1. Jacobson JA. Chapter 1, Introduction. In: Fundamentals of Musculoskeletal Ultrasound. Saunders W.B.; 2017
2. Ziegler DW. The use of in-office, orthopaedist-performed ultrasound of the shoulder to evaluate and manage rotator cuff disorders. J Shoulder Elbow Surg 2004;13(3):291–297
3. Al-Shawi A, Badge R, Bunker T. The detection of full thickness rotator cuff tears using ultrasound. J Bone Joint Surg Br 2008;90(7):889–892
4. Roy JS, Braën C, Leblond J, et al. Diagnostic accuracy of ultrasonography, MRI and MR arthrography in the characterisation of rotator cuff disorders: a systematic review and meta-analysis. Br J Sports Med 2015;49(20):1316–1328
5. Iannotti JP, Ciccone J, Buss DD, et al. Accuracy of office-based ultrasonography of the shoulder for the diagnosis of rotator cuff tears. J Bone Joint Surg Am 2005;87(6):1305–1311
6. Teefey SA, Hasan SA, Middleton WD, Patel M, Wright RW, Yamaguchi K. Ultrasonography of the rotator cuff: a comparison of ultrasonographic and arthroscopic findings in one hundred consecutive cases. J Bone Joint Surg Am 2000;82(4):498–504
7. de Jesus, Parker L, Frangos AJ, Nazarian LN. Accuracy of MRI, MR arthrography, and ultrasound in the diagnosis of rotator cuff tears: a meta-analysis. AJR Am J Roentgenol 2009;192(6):1701–1707
8. Prickett WD, Teefey SA, Galatz LM, Calfee RP, Middleton WD, Yamaguchi K. Accuracy of ultrasound imaging of the rotator cuff in shoulders that are painful postoperatively. J Bone Joint Surg Am 2003;85(6):1084–1089
9. Alavekios DA, Dionysian E, Sodl J, Contreras R, Cho Y, Yian EH. Longitudinal analysis of effects of operator experience on accuracy for ultrasound detection of supraspinatus tears. J Shoulder Elbow Surg 2013;22(3):375–380
10. Murphy RJ, Daines MT, Carr AJ, Rees JL. An independent learning method for orthopaedic surgeons performing shoulder ultrasound to identify full-thickness tears of the rotator cuff. J Bone Joint Surg Am 2013;95(3):266–272

Suggested Reading

Jacobson JA. Chapter 3, Shoulder ultrasound. In: Fundamentals of Musculoskeletal Ultrasound. Saunders W.B.; 2017

7 Diagnostic and Therapeutic Injections

Suresh K. Nayar and Uma Srikumaran

Summary

Injections may be used both as a diagnostic aid and to provide therapeutic relief for common acromioclavicular, glenohumeral, rotator cuff, biceps, and suprascapular shoulder pathologies.

Keywords: Injection, therapeutic, diagnostic, pain relief, imaging

I. General overview

A. Injections can be diagnostic to determine source of pain/injury or therapeutic to provide temporary relief:

1. Diagnostic for:

   a. Acromioclavicular (AC) joint pathology

   b. Rotator cuff tears

   c. Subacromial impingement

   d. Anterolateral pain syndrome

   e. Glenohumeral joint pathology

   f. Suprascapular nerve entrapment

   g. Biceps tendon pathology.

2. Therapeutic injections:

   a. Provides pain relief for multiple conditions, including but not limited to: osteoarthritis, rheumatoid arthritis, adhesive capsulitis, calcific tendinitis, rotator cuff tears, subacromial bursitis, biceps tendinitis, and impingement

   b. To be used after other conservative therapies (nonsteroidal anti-inflammatory drugs [NSAIDs], physical therapy, disease-modifying agents for rheumatoid arthritis) have failed

   c. Typically a combination of corticosteroid and anesthetic

   d. Immediate relief suggests drug is delivered accurately to site of pain

   e. Relief in hours or days is reflective of systemic absorption of corticosteroid

   f. May see relief for up to 6 months

   g. May receive not more than three to four injections per year:

      i. Avoid repeat injections for biceps tendon pathology to avoid risk of rupture.

   h. Can aid in adjunctive physical therapy (e.g., calcific tendinitis):

      i. See ▶Table 7.1 for commonly used preparations.

Table 7.1 Commonly used preparations for therapeutic shoulder injections

Site	Syringe (in mL)	Anesthetic* (in mL)	Corticosteroid** (in mL)
Acromioclavicular joint	3 to 5	0.5	0.25 to 0.5
Subacromial space	10	5 to 7	1 to 2
Glenohumeral joint	10	5 to 7	1 to 2
Biceps tendon area	3 to 5	0.5	0.25
Scapulothoracic articulation	3 to 5	1 to 2	0.5 to 1.0

Notes: *1% lidocaine or 0.25 to 0.5% bupivacaine.
**Betamethasone sodium phosphate and acetate (Celestone Soluspan) or methylprednisolone (Depo-Medrol, 40 mg/mL) or triamcinolone acetonide (Kenalog, 40 mg/mL).
Recommend a 21 to 25 cc gauge needle, 1.5 inches, depending on site of injection.

B. Technique:
1. Accuracy may be improved with ultrasound guidance
2. Performed with sterile technique and consistent pressure
3. Aspiration before injection avoids intravascular injection
4. Agent should flow freely when injected into articular space
5. Anesthetic injection in overlying soft tissue with a 25 gauge needle is optional
6. Passive manipulation after injection aids in dispersion of the therapeutic
7. Patient should be monitored in office for up to half an hour following injection
8. Avoid strenuous activity for at least 48 hours following injection.

C. Contraindications:
1. Absolute:
   a. Suspected infection
   b. Prosthetic joint
   c. Intratendinous injections.
2. Relative:
   a. Prior adverse reaction
   b. Active skin lesions at site of injection
   c. Anticoagulant use or elevated international normalized ratio (INR).

D. Complications and side effects
1. Skin atrophy or depigmentation of injection site
2. Postinjection flare from crystal deposition, generally resolves in 48 hours
3. Infection occurs rarely (1:2,000 to 1:20,000 injections), typically begins after 48 hours
4. Single intra-articular injections have negligible effects on glycemic control

5. Soft tissue injection or peri-tendinous injections may elevate blood glu-
cose (from 5 to 21 days) and may require closer glycemic monitoring.

E. There are no studies showing lasting benefit from platelet enriched plasma
injections for shoulder pathology

F. Diagnosis of shoulder pathology is made from a combination of physical examination, imaging, and injection.

II. Acromioclavicular joint pathology

A. Physical examination findings are more accurate and reliable for AC joint pathology compared to rotator cuff injury due to accessibility of joint

B. Smaller joint with fibrous capsule makes injections more challenging with accurate
intra-articular needle placement ranging from 39 to 67%

C. Peri-articular and intra-articular injections may be equally efficacious

D. Technique:
  1. Palpate distal end of clavicle and move laterally until a soft spot is
  encountered

  2. Orient needle vertically in a cephalad to caudal direction with a slight,
  5 degrees, inward tilt (▶Fig. 7.1)

  3. Passing the needle too deeply may inject agent into the subacromial space
  which should be avoided

  4. If using ultrasound, having the patient flex elbow and place hand over contralateral shoulder may stress the AC joint and show instability, if present.

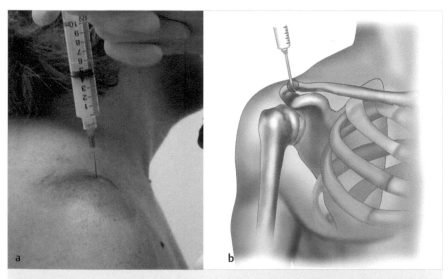

Fig. 7.1 (a, b) Needle orientation, anatomy, and approach of each injection for acromioclavicular
(AC), subacromial (anterior, lateral, and posterior), glenohumeral (anterior and posterior),
suprascapular, and biceps tendon injections.

III. Rotator cuff and subacromial space pathology

A. Rotator cuff injury results from intrinsic (degeneration) and extrinsic (impingement, trauma) causes

B. Subacromial bursal fibers typically contain highest density of painful nerve fibers

C. Most useful physical examination findings are weakness with resisted abduction or external rotation, drop-arm sign, external rotation lag sign, and painful arc of motion

D. Because physical examination and imaging are often equivocal, therapeutic and diagnostic injections have high utility

E. Accuracy ranges from 56 to 92%

F. Given the ease of access to subacromial space, ultrasound guidance is not typically needed, but may help see bursal distension with accurate needle placement

G. Must avoid injecting directly into rotator cuff

H. Technique (▶ **Fig. 7.1**):
   1. Patient should be seated, allowing the arm to hang freely at the side or rest in the patient's lap:
       a. Anterior:
           i. Least recommended due to coracoacromial ligament and/or anterior acromial spurs
           ii. Palpate for soft spot between inferior border of anterolateral acromion and humeral head.
       b. Lateral:
           i. Most preferred
           ii. Palpate for soft spot between inferior border of posterior-third lateral acromion and greater tuberosity
           iii. Direct needle to contralateral nipple.
       c. Posterior:
           i. Recommended when pain is primarily posterior
           ii. Palpate for soft spot just inferior to posterolateral aspect of acromion.

IV. Glenohumeral joint

A. Co-existing disorders, such as, biceps tendon pathology, superior labral anterior to posterior (SLAP) and rotator cuff tears, chondral lesions, adhesive capsulitis, and impingement, may confound source of pain

B. Radiography may be superior to injection in diagnosing arthritis

C. Accuracy ranges from 50 to >90%, improve with ultrasound

D. Technique:

1. Two approaches with patient seated:

   a. Anterior (▶ **Fig. 7.1**):

      i. While moving the arm through external and internal rotations when adducted at the patient's side, palpate anteriorly for the rotator cuff interval which is lateral (~1 cm) and just superior to the coracoid

      ii. Direct needle posteriorly with slight superolateral tilt to parallel glenoid version

      iii. If the humeral head is felt to be moving after seating the needle, redirect medially

      iv. If the needle hits bone and there is no appreciable movement, it is likely resting on the glenoid and needs to be redirected laterally.

   b. Posterior (▶ **Fig. 7.1**):

      i. Palpate for soft spot just inferior (~2 cm) and medial (~1 cm) to posterolateral corner of acromion and aim toward coracoid.

V. Suprascapular nerve

A. Pathology secondary to traction (overhead activity) or compressive (synovial or ganglion cyst, ▶ **Fig. 7.2**) injury affecting the suprascapular nerve at the scapular notch or spinoglenoid notch

B. Suprascapular nerve injury affects both supraspinatus and infraspinatus

C. Spinoglenoid notch compression affects infraspinatus only

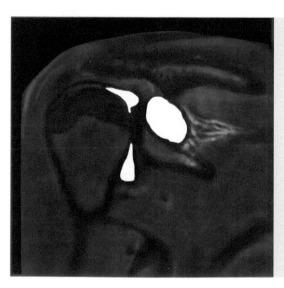

Fig. 7.2 Imaging depicting spinoglenoid cyst.

D. Injection typically performed after electromyography studies:

    1. Technique:

        a. Recommend fluoroscopic or ultrasound guidance to avoid nerve injury or vascular insult.

VI. Biceps tendon

A. Associated pain is often ambiguous and can mimic other pathologies, including osteoarthritis, rotator cuff injury, and AC joint pain

B. Biceps injury often co exists with another pathology

C. Most physical examination findings are less reliable

D. Poor accuracy without ultrasound guidance (~27 versus 87% with guidance)

E. Injections can also enter glenohumeral space through tendon sheath proximally, complicating diagnostic utility

F. Technique:

    1. With the patient supine, flex elbow to 90 degrees and externally rotate shoulder 20 degrees to move tendon away from anterior joint line

    2. Locate tendon with ultrasound (▶ Fig. 7.3), and avoid injecting directly into the tendon

    3. Injecting without ultrasound assistance is not recommended; if needed, however, palpate for the maximal point of tenderness and feel for the moving tendon at the proximal humerus as the elbow is ranged

    4. Direct needle ~30 degrees medially and parallel to groove.

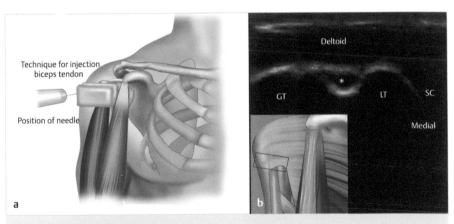

Fig. 7.3 (a, b) Illustration and ultrasound image showing location for biceps tendon injection. GT, greater tuberosity; LT, lesser tuberosity; *, biceps tendon; SC, subscapularis.

Suggested Readings

McFarland E, Bernard J, Dein E, Johnson A. Diagnostic injections about the shoulder. J Am Acad Orthop Surg 2017;25(12):799–807

Skedros JG, Hunt KJ, Pitts TC. Variations in corticosteroid/anesthetic injections for painful shoulder conditions: comparisons among orthopaedic surgeons, rheumatologists, and physical medicine and primary-care physicians. BMC Musculoskelet Disord 2007;8:63

Tallia AF, Cardone DA. Diagnostic and therapeutic injection of the shoulder region. Am Fam Physician 2003;67(6):1271–1278

8 Rotator Cuff Disease

Ankit Bansal and Uma Srikumaran

Summary

Rotator cuff disease is a highly prevalent phenomenon in patients >40 years old. It is a continuum of disease, where acute trauma or chronic damage can lead to rotator cuff tears and eventual arthropathy. This chapter outlines the epidemiology, pathophysiology, clinical presentation, and treatment options of rotator cuff tears.

Keywords: Rotator cuff tear, continuum, prevalence, diagnosis, management

I. Overview

A. Continuum of disease: Subacromial or subcoracoid impingement, calcific tendonitis, partial- or full-thickness rotator cuff (RTC) tears, massive tears, and cuff tear arthropathy.

II. Epidemiology

A. Prevalence: 7–40% in cadaveric studies

B. Age >60: 28% have full-thickness tear

C. Age >70: 65% have full-thickness tear

D. In those with unilateral painful full-thickness tears, there is 56% chance of having an asymptomatic contralateral full- or partial-thickness tear

E. Of all asymptomatic tears, 50% will get symptoms in 3 years. Of these, 40% will have progression of tear.

III. Pathophysiology

A. Chronic degenerative tear:
    1. Seen in older patients
    2. Most commonly involves the supraspinatus and infraspinatus
    3. Can extend to subscapularis and teres minor
    4. Attributed to age-related intrinsic degeneration of the tendon
    5. Disoriented collagen fibers, myxoid, and hyaline degeneration.

B. Chronic impingement:
    1. Typically starts at bursal surface of supraspinatus and infraspinatus
    2. Os acromiale or bony acromial spur causes direct pressure and attritional injury to the bursal tendon
    3. Deteriorated scapular motion most common cause of extrinsic RTC tearing
    4. Also seen in internal impingement in overhead throwing athletes:

      a.   Partial articular supraspinatus tendon avulsion (PASTA) tears seen from impingement of posterosuperior glenoid and articular RTC.

C.   Acute traumatic avulsions:

    1.   Seen with shoulder dislocations in age >40 years

    2.   Subscapularis avulsions seen in younger patients from hyperabduction/external rotation injuries

    3.   Acute avulsion may have better prognosis than chronic degenerative tear, if repaired in the acute phase.

D.   Iatrogenic:

    1.   Subscapularis failure seen after open anterior shoulder surgery from failure of repair.

IV. Anatomy

A.   Five layers:

    1.   Layer I: Most superficial thin layer, composed of fibers from coracohumeral ligament

    2.   Layer II: Dense collage fibers parallel to long axis of tendon (3–5 mm thick)

    3.   Layer III: Smaller loose bundles of collagen at 45 degrees angle to Layer II (3 mm thick)

    4.   Layer IV: Loose connective tissue continuous with coracohumeral ligament

    5.   Layer V: Shoulder capsule (2 mm thick).

B.   Articular-side fibers have only half the strength of bursal side

C.   Rotator interval:

    1.   Located in between supraspinatus and subscapularis

    2.   Comprises superior glenohumeral ligament (SGHL), coracohumeral ligament, long head of biceps tendon, and capsule.

D.   Rotator cable:

    1.   Runs perpendicularly along the insertions of supraspinatus and infraspinatus

    2.   Thick fibers at the avascular zone of the coracohumeral ligament.

V. Classification

A.   Cuff tear size (DeOrio and Cofield):

    1.   Small: Less than 1 cm

    2.   Medium: 1–3 cm

    3.   Large: 3–5 cm

    4.   Massive: ILrger than 5 cm (multiple tendons).

B.   Partial-thickness RTC tears (Ellman):

    1.   Grade I (<3 mm, <25% thickness), Grade II (3–6 mm, 25–50%), Grade III (>6 mm, >50%)

    2.   A – Articular sided, B – Bursal sided, C – Intratendinous.

C. Cuff atrophy (Goutallier grade)

1. 0–Normal
2. 1–Some fatty streaks
3. 2–More muscle than fat
4. 3–Equal amounts of fat and muscle
5. 4–More fat than muscle.

D. Cuff tear shape (▶ **Fig. 8.1**)–Site Burkhart: Crescent, U-shape, L-shape, massive and immobile.

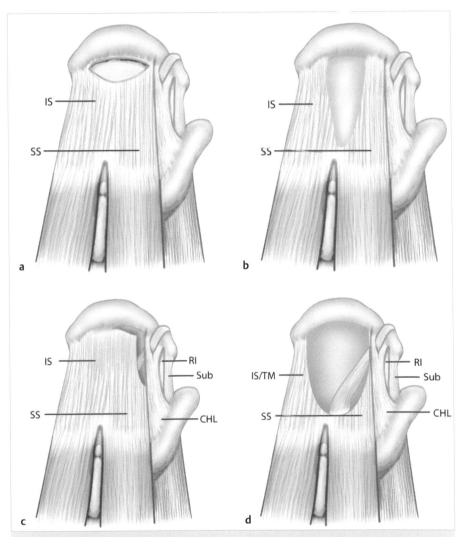

Fig. 8.1 (a) Crescent-shaped tear. (b) U-shaped tear. (c) L-shaped tear. (d) Massive contracted tear.

VI. Presentation

A. Insidious onset of pain with overhead activities

B. Night pain, deltoid pain, lateral humeral pain, and muscular weakness

C. Common to have active and passive range of motion (ROM) differences

D. Acute development of pain after trauma could indicate traumatic rupture

E. Physical examination:

    1. Impingement: Hawkin's test, Neer's test

    2. Supraspinatus tear: Jobe's test, drop arm test

    3. Infraspinatus tear: External rotation (ER) test at 0 degrees abduction, ER lag sign

    4. Teres minor tear: Hornblower's sign

    5. Subscapularis tear: Belly press test, lift off test, excessive passive ER.

F. Important to assess postural alignment and scapular mechanics

G. Positive shrug sign and stiffness

H. Imaging and examination findings don't always correlate, and it is the surgeon's responsibility to reconcile the differences.

VII. Imaging

A. Radiographs:

    1. Anteroposterior (AP), Grashey (true AP), internal and external rotations, axillary lateral, and scapular Y views

    2. Greater tuberosity cystic changes, acromial spurring, calcific tendonitis, proximal humeral migration (<7 mm acromiohumeral interval), secondary arthrosis, and type III hooked acromion (▶Fig. 8.2)

B. Magnetic resonance imaging (MRI):

    1. Standard of care for diagnosis of RTC pathology (▶Fig. 8.2)

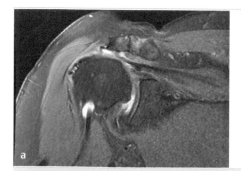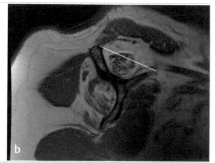

Fig. 8.2 MRI cuff tear, tangent sign classification. **(a)** Coronal MRI showing full thickness, full width, retracted supraspinatus tear. **(b)** Sagittal MRI showing Goutallier grade IV rotator cuff atrophy. Muscle belly lies below the tangent line (drawn laterally from superior aspect of scapular spine medially to superior aspect of coracoid).

2. Determine size, shape, type, and degree of tendon retraction or delamination
3. Assess degree of muscle atrophy (Goutallier classification):
   a. Tangent sign (▶**Fig. 8.2**)—indicative of severe irreparable supraspinatus atrophy.
4. Greater tuberosity cystic changes in chronic RTC disease
5. Assess labrum, chondral damage, and associated arthritic conditions
6. Assess biceps subluxation, indicative of subscapularis tear
7. Assess for bone marrow edema within greater tuberosity and acromion
8. Assess acromioclavicular joint and subacromial bursa.

C. Ultrasound:
1. Advantages:
   a. Dynamic examination
   b. Immediate assessment of suspected RTC tear
   c. Inexpensive
   d. Repeat examination following repair
   e. Useful for localizing injections.
2. Disadvantages:
   a. User dependent
   b. Limited utility for evaluating associated intra-articular pathology.
3. Sensitivity/Specificity:
   a. Sensitivity, specificity, and overall accuracy for diagnosis of RTC disease is comparable to MRI.

VIII. Management considerations

A. Age and activity demands
B. Mode of failure for RTC (degenerative or acute traumatic)
C. Tear morphology:
1. Avulsion versus muscle–tendon junction
2. Partial- versus full-thickness tear
3. Articular-sided (PASTA lesion) versus bursal-sided tear.
D. Surgical approach:
1. Arthroscopic versus mini-open
2. Repair versus debridement
3. Massive RTC tear: Partial repair versus graft augmentation versus capsular reconstruction.

IX. Natural history

A. 51% of previously asymptomatic RTC tears became symptomatic at mean of 2.8 years
B. Nearly half the patients younger than 60 years had progression of previously known full-thickness RTC tear

C. Clinical progression of symptoms correlated with tear progression and fatty infiltration

D. Fatty infiltration (Goutallier Grade 2) occurred at an average of 3 years after known supraspinatus tear; Grade 3 occurred at an average of 5 years

E. Positive tangent sign appeared at an average of 4.5 years after onset of symptoms

F. Nonoperative management of massive RTC tears maintained satisfactory shoulder function for 4 years before significant degenerative structural changes.

X. Nonoperative treatment

A. Indications:
   1. Asymptomatic RTC tear
   2. First line of treatment for most tears
   3. Elderly low-demand patient
   4. Medical contraindications to surgery
   5. RTC arthropathy.

B. Technique:
   1. Activity modifications, avoid overhead painful movements
   2. Oral anti-inflammatory medications
   3. Oral short-course steroid tapers
   4. Physical therapy:
      a. Largely to maintain functional ROM
      b. Avoid heavy strengthening workouts, as this may result in progression of symptoms.
   5. Steroid injections:
      a. Subacromial for impingement, bursal-sided tears, and bursitis
      b. Glenohumeral for associated synovitis and stiffness.

XI. Operative treatment

A. Indications:
   1. Acute full-thickness RTC tears
   2. Chronic full-thickness RTC tear failing conservative treatment:
      a. Patients should be counseled that a persistently torn RTC will progress, but may remain asymptomatic.
   3. Symptomatic partial RTC tears:
      a. Bursal-sided tears >3 mm (>25%)
      b. Articular-sided tears >6 mm (>50%)
      c. In situ fixation of acute traumatic injuries
      d. Completion and repair of chronic degenerative tendons.

B. Techniques, outcomes, and rehabilitation:
   1. See next chapter.

XII. Subscapularis tear

A. Anatomy:
   1. Subscapularis is the only anterior muscle of all RTC tendons
   2. Strong dynamic stabilizer and powerful internal rotator
   3. Contributes to the force couple in the coronal and transverse planes
   4. Multiple intra-muscular tendons present
   5. The proximal aspect of subscapularis has the broadest insertion, and is the most tendinous in nature. It inserts onto the fovea capitis of the proximal humerus. This is the most critical part of the muscle unit, and can be visualized intra-articularly.

B. Pathophysiology:
   1. Subcoracoid impingement from the roller-wringer effect:
      a. Impingement of coracoid process and proximal humerus in forward flexion 120–130 degrees and internal rotation of the arm
      b. Less than 7 mm between coracoid process and humerus is abnormal.
   2. Usually involves the superior edge of the tendon
   3. Can result from severe anterior instability
   4. Iatrogenic injury following surgical manipulation (tenotomy, peel, split).

C. Presentation:
   1. Liftoff test, Belly press sign, and Bearhug sign (see points listed under physical examination, section VI Presentation)
   2. Increased external rotation
   3. Biceps subluxation on axial MRI is pathognomonic for subscapularis tear:
      a. Indicates tear of transverse humeral ligament and violation of bicipital sling.
   4. Arthroscopy can identify a comma sign:
      a. Represents avulsed SGHL and coracohumeral ligament (comma tissue).

D. Surgical treatment:
   1. Either open or arthroscopic repair
   2. Reduce subcoracoid impingement with partial resection of coracoid process
   3. Pectoralis major tendon transfer for chronic tears and deficiencies.

9 Arthroscopic Rotator Cuff Repair: Single-Row, Double-Row, and Transosseous-Equivalent Repair

Paul S. Ragusa, Ankit Bansal, and Uma Srikumaran

Summary

The goal of rotator cuff repair is to obtain secure, tension-free fixation of the tendon to the anatomic footprint. Arthroscopic techniques include single-row (SR), double-row (DR), and transosseous-equivalent (TOE) repair. Several biomechanical studies have shown superiority of DR and TOE repair over SR repair. Despite biomechanical superiority of DR over SR repair, clinical outcomes have not found any significant difference between the two techniques at short-term follow-up. Consistent with biomechanical outcomes, retear rates are lower for DR repair than SR repair; however, the clinical relevance of a rotator cuff retear remains controversial.

Keywords: Rotator cuff, single-row repair, double-row repair, transosseous-equivalent repair, retear rate, biomechanical outcomes, clinical outcomes

I. Introduction

A. The goal of rotator cuff repair is to obtain secure, tension-free fixation of the tendon to the anatomic footprint so that biologic tendon-to-bone healing can occur

B. Open transosseous rotator cuff repair had been considered the gold standard technique, and has performed well in clinical and biomechanical studies

C. The transition from open to arthroscopic repair has brought about an evolution of techniques that include single- and double-row constructs, and more recently transosseous-equivalent (TOE) or suture-bridge repair

D. The optimal technique is still controversial and the superiority of one construct over another is not well established.

II. Single-row (SR) repair

A. SR repair (▶ **Fig. 9.1a**) of a full-thickness rotator cuff tear utilizes a linear row of suture anchors (typically double- and/or triple-loaded) inserted into the medial or lateral aspect of the rotator cuff footprint depending on tendon mobility

B. Suture anchors inserted at 90 degrees to the surface of the rotator cuff footprint have been shown to have less gap formation and increased cyclic load to failure when compared to those inserted at the "deadman's angle" of 45 degrees[1]

C. Suture limbs are passed through the tendon in a variety of suture configurations (simple, mattress, modified Mason-Allen, etc.)

D. The advantages of this technique are that it is easy, quick, and does not require a large amount of residual tendon length.

E. SR repair is recommended in tears where there is <1 cm of remnant tendon length[2]

F. Most published data suggest that an SR repair is sufficient for small and medium sized rotator cuff tears (<3 cm).[3]

III. Double-row (DR) repair

A. DR repair (▶Fig. 9.1b) was introduced by Lo and Burkhart in 2003[4]

B. DR repair involves placing a medial row of suture anchors along the humeral head articular margin and a second row of anchors on the lateral aspect of the footprint

C. Suture limbs from the medial row are passed 5 mm distal to the musculotendinous junction in a mattress configuration; lateral row sutures may be passed in a simple or mattress configuration

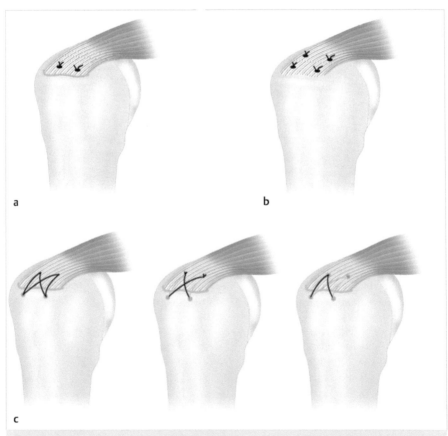

Fig. 9.1 Illustration of different rotator cuff repair constructs. (a) Single-row (SR) anchor repair. (b) Double-row (DR) suture anchor repair; (c) Transosseous-equivalent (TOE) repair; for TOE repair, the medial row sutures can be knotted (left) or knotless (right).

D. Care must be taken to avoid excessive tensioning of the repair; this can be achieved by ensuring that adequate tendon length and excursion are available

E. An advantage of this technique over SR repair is that it is biomechanically superior and provides improved footprint restoration which theoretically allows a greater surface area for tendon-to-bone healing to occur

F. Disadvantages of this technique include increased operating room time, increased difficulty, and anchor crowding in the footprint

G. Most published data suggest that DR repair may be preferable for large and massive tears with adequate tendon length[3]

H. Significant tissue loss or remnant tissue on the lateral footprint precludes the use of a DR repair.

IV. Transosseous-equivalent (TOE) repair

A. TOE (▶ Fig. 9.1c) was introduced by Park et al. in 2006

B. TOE repair, also known as a suture-bridge repair, is a modification of the DR repair where the medial row suture limbs are linked to knotless anchors on the lateral humeral cortex; this differs from the DR repair where each suture anchor acts as a separate point of fixation

C. Passage of medial row sutures through the musculotendinous junction should be avoided because of the risk of medial row failure[5]

D. Since the lateral anchors are inserted in the lateral cortex, it avoids the problem of suture anchor crowing in the footprint seen with DR repair

E. Another advantage is that it provides a broader surface area of contact similar to transosseous repair; this differs from the "spot-weld" fixation seen with DR repair

F. A major disadvantage to using this technique is that the vascular supply to the tendon may be compromised by the increased pressure over the bursal side of the tendon.

V. Biomechanical outcomes

A. The biomechanical properties necessary to achieve successful rotator cuff repair include a high initial fixation strength (measured as ultimate load to failure), minimum gap formation at the time of repair, maintenance of mechanical stability under cyclic loading, and optimization of the biology of the tendon–bone interface until healing occurs

B. Several technical parameters have been used to effect rotator cuff repair strength including modifying suture anchor configuration, modifying suture configuration (i.e., simple suture, mattress suture, modified Mason-Allen, etc.), and altering the number and type of sutures used

C. Several biomechanical studies have shown superiority of DR to SR repair with regard to mechanical strength,[6–8] footprint coverage,[9] and gap formation[6]

D.   TOE repair has been shown to be superior to DR repair by providing a larger area of contact pressure[10] and higher ultimate-to-load failure[11]

E.   A recent systematic review of 40 biomechanical studies found that the type of suture and the number of suture limbs that pass through the tendon may be stronger predictors of fixation strength than the construct type:[12]

   1.   Four major findings were revealed:[12]

      a.   The number of suture limbs passed through the tendon may be a stronger predictor of ultimate failure load than the number of sutures used

      b.   Although TOE repair achieved the highest ultimate load to failure, no significant difference was found between repair types when stratified by the total number of suture limbs that passed through the tendon

      c.   A higher number of suture limbs that passed through the tendon and the use of TOE repair increased the risk of developing a type 2 retear

      d.   Using wide sutures instead of standard sutures correlated with higher failure load.

VI. Functional outcomes

A.   Several Level I randomized controlled trials (RCTs) evaluating clinical outcomes after SR and DR repairs have not found any significant difference between the two techniques at short-term follow-up[13–17]

B.   In addition, several recent meta-analyses have also reported no difference in clinical outcomes between SR and DR repairs[18–20]

C.   However, there is some evidence to suggest clinical superiority of DR repair over SR repair when performed for larger tears

D.   A Level I RCT of 160 patients with a full-thickness rotator cuff tear found superior clinical outcomes at 2 years with DR repair compared to SR repair, especially for tears >3 cm[21]

E.   A Level II cohort study of 78 patients with a full-thickness rotator cuff tear >3 cm found significantly improved subjective outcomes (Constant and American Shoulder and Elbow Surgeons [ASES] scores) at 2 years after DR repair when compared to SR repair; however, no significant differences between techniques were found when all tear sizes were included[22]

F.   A Level II RCT of 53 patients with an initial tear size of >3 cm in sagittal length underwent SR and DR repairs with a minimum 2-year follow-up. The patients with initial tears >3 cm in sagittal length had improved strength at 2 years when treated with DR repair compared with SR repair[23]

G.   Two recent meta-analyses also indicate potentially better clinical outcomes with DR repairs in patients with a tear size >3 cm[24,25]

H.   Although there are several studies which show successful clinical outcomes with TOE repair, there are no studies that show superior clinical outcomes of this technique over others.[26–30]

VII. Structural outcomes

A. The incidence of retear after rotator cuff repair varies widely in the literature

B. Historical estimates range from 11% to as high as 94% in patients with large and massive tears[31–39]

C. A classic study using ultrasound to evaluate cuff integrity found a retear incidence of 94% after SR repair of tears measuring >2 cm[31]

D. Patient's age, initial tear size, and fatty degeneration of the supraspinatus are independent risk factors for a rotator cuff retear[40]

E. The clinical relevance of a rotator cuff retear remains controversial; although some studies suggest that repair integrity does not affect clinical outcomes,[41–43] several studies have shown that retears affect functional scores[44–49]

F. Consistent with biomechanical outcomes, multiple systematic reviews and meta-analyses have reported that retear rates are lower for DR repair compared to SR repair[18,19,24,50,51]

G. Similarly, studies have shown superior healing rates for TOE repair compared to SR repair, particularly for larger and massive tears;[49,51–54] however, the retear rates of small tears <1 cm do not appear to differ between TOE and SR techniques[50,51]

H. To date, no Level I study has shown that TOE technique yields superior healing rates compared with conventional DR repair; a recent systematic review found that retear rates for DR and TOE repairs did not differ significantly from each other in any tear size category.

VIII. Retear pattern

A. Two patterns of rotator cuff retear have been described[55] (▶Fig. 9.2)

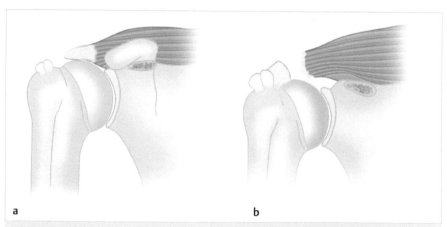

a   b

Fig. 9.2 Illustration of two different patterns of rotator retear. (a) Type 1 Retear: Failure of the tendon occurs at the site of repair, often with tendon detachment from the bone. (b) Type 2 Retear: Failure occurs medial to the repair at the muscle–tendon junction with remnants of the tendon still attached to the bone.

B. Type 1 failure occurs when the tendon fails to heal and detaches at the site of repair often with tendon detachment from the bone:

    1. The weakest part of a suture anchor repair construct is at the suture–tendon interface, and the most common mode of failure is suture cutout through the tendon.[3]

C. Type 2 failure occurs when the tendon fails medial to the repair at the muscle–tendon junction with remnants of the tendon still attached to the bone:

    1. The mechanism of failure of type 2 retears has been attributed to tension overload at the musculotendinous junction of the supraspinatus[12]

    2. Type 2 failures are associated with a worse prognosis than type 1 failures.[56]

D. Retear patterns are similar depending on the method of rotator cuff repair:

    1. Type 1 retears are typically seen after SR repair

    2. Type 2 retears are typically seen after TOE repairs and DR repairs:[55,57]

        a. Several studies suggest that excessive tissue contact pressure and tension overload in the medial row of TOE repairs cause strangulation of micro-circulation resulting in reduced blood supply to the tendon[58–60]

        b. Recent studies suggest that the TOE repair construct alone may not be responsible for the type 2 retear pattern, and techniques used to decrease overtensioning at the musculotendinous junction such as leaving the medial row sutures untied[61] or using rapidly absorbable sutures for the medial row[62] may lead to lower rates of type 2 failure.

E. Revision surgery in the setting of a type 2 tear is difficult, and options are limited compared with type 1 tears:

    1. Revision options for a type 2 retear are likely to rely on tendon-to-tendon healing, whereas type 1 retears do not result in the loss of tendon stock and can be repaired again to the anatomic footprint.[63]

IX. Conclusion

A. The goal of rotator cuff repair is to obtain secure, tension-free fixation of the tendon to the anatomic footprint so that biologic tendon-to-bone healing can occur

B. Arthroscopic techniques include SR, DR, and TOE repair. The optimal technique is still controversial and the superiority of one construct over another is not well established

C. Several biomechanical studies have shown superiority of DR and TOE repairs over SR repair with respect to mechanical strength, footprint coverage, tendon-to-bone contact pressure and gap formation

D. A recent systematic review of these biomechanical studies found that modifying the number of sutures, suture limbs, and mattress stitches in a construct are stronger predictors of fixation strength than the construct type

E. Despite biomechanical superiority of DR repair over SR repair, several Level I RCTs evaluating clinical outcomes have not found any significant difference between the two techniques at short-term follow-up

F. Some studies suggest superior clinical outcomes with DR repair compared to SR repair for tears >3 cm

G. Consistent with biomechanical outcomes, multiple systematic reviews and meta-analyses have reported that retear rates are lower for DR repair compared with SR repair; however, the clinical relevance of a rotator cuff retear remains controversial

H. Type 2 retears are typically seen after TOE repairs and have been attributed to tension overload at the musculotendinous junction of the supraspinatus; increased construct strength of TOE repair needs to be balanced with the higher risk of these type 2 failure.

X. Subscapularis repairs

A. Lafosse classification of subscapularis tears and treatment algorithm [64]

B. Recommended order of steps:[65]

1. Perform diagnostic arthroscopy

2. Address biceps, tenotomy vs. tenodesis

3. Establish a window through the rotator interval

4. If adhesions present, perform skeletanization of the posterolateral coracoid and perform a 3-sided release of the subscapularis tendon

5. Perform coracoidplasty if indicated (<7 mm coracohumeral distance)

6. Lesser tuberosity bone bed preparation

7. Repair remainder of rotator cuff.

C. Use anterosuperolateral (ASL) portal for instrumentation

D. Access subcoracoid space using 30 degree arthroscope. The coracoid is present just anterior to the upper subscapularis

E. Free adhesions to tendon posteriorly off the glenoid rim and anteriorly through surrounding fascia

F. Beware of excessive medial dissection anterior to subscapularis due to neurovascular structures

G. Traction suture or grasper may be useful to assess reduction to native footprint

H. Preparing footprint involves electrocautery and bone burring to create healthy bone bed

I. The normal medial margin of the subscapularis is 2–3 mm lateral to the articular margin. The lateral margin is marked by the bicipital groove

J. In cases of low tendon excursion, it may be reasonable to place footprint up to the edge of the articular cartilage. In severe cases, further medialization is an option with no observed decrease in functional outcomes

K. Various suture configurations can be used to repair the tendon:

1. Horizontal mattress

2. Simple suture

3. Single-row vs. Double-row

4. Knotless vs. Knot anchors.

L. If performing intra-articular biceps tenodesis, surgeon may use that anchor and lateral row fixation of subscapularis repair

M. Open repair can be performed via deltopectoral approach in cases of large isolated subscapularis tears

N. For irreparable tears, in the absence of glenohumeral arthritis in the younger population, allograft augmentation and anterior capsular reconstruction may be utilized. Pectoralis major and latissimus dorsi transfers have also been described

O. Reverse shoulder arthroplasty is the best salvage operation in chronic failures.

XI. Rehabilitation after rotator cuff repair

A. General principles:

1. The goal of rotator cuff surgery and rehabilitation is to return the patient to their optimal functional improvement

2. A successful rehabilitation program implements exercises that restore optimal function while protecting anatomic integrity of injured or repaired tissue

3. The exercises should allow progression of intensity and load within healing tissues capability

4. The strength of a successfully repaired rotator cuff tendon is 30% that of a normal tendon after six weeks, 52% after three months, and 81% after six months[66]

5. Anatomic failure is associated with increasing age, poor tissue quality, fatty infiltration, atrophy, smoking, hypercholesterolemia, and diabetes; it tends to occur in the first 3–6 months after surgery.

B. Timing of therapy depends on the patient, the tear, and the quality of the repair:

1. Protected passive range of motion (PROM) should be considered during the first 6 weeks after arthroscopic rotator cuff repair of small to medium tears (< 4 cm)

2. A 6-week period of strict immobilization with delayed start of PROM activities should be considered if there are concerns regarding tissue healing

3. Patients at risk for stiffness (diabetes, thyroid disorders, acute rotator cuff tears, partial-thickness tears, and adhesive capsulitis) may benefit from additional focus on their PROM during the first 6 weeks

4. Excessive early activity:

    a. Produces pain

    b. Increases tensile loads

    c. Can increase the inflammatory response

    d. Raises concern for retearing or detachment of the RTC repair.

5. Insufficient activity may lead to:

    a. Decreased motion

    b. Joint adhesions

    c. Decreased muscle activation.

C. Supervised rehabilitation should monitor external rotation in neutral abduction and forward elevation ROM as indicators of progress

D. One rehabilitation program is not drastically better than the next provided they follow a logical and progressive return to activity

1. Phase I (First 4 weeks of therapy):

    a. Typically begins 4–6 weeks after surgery

    b. Goals: Patient education and passive range of motion with minimal pain

    c. Patient education: posture, joint protection, positioning, and hygiene

    d. Elbow, wrist, and hand AROM without weight

        i. Only PROM of elbow if biceps tenodesis was performed.

    e. Passive forward elevation to 90 degrees

    f. Passive external rotation (elbow at side) to 30 degrees

    g. Only PROM activities with low rotator cuff EMG activity (i.e. no pulleys, cane exercises, or self PROM)

    h. Begin active and manual scapula strengthening exercises.

2. Phase II (Weeks 5 to 7):

    a. Goal: Gradual progression of PROM

    b. Progress scapula strengthening

    c. Progress passive forward elevation and passive external rotation

    d. May begin aquatic therapy after 6 weeks for active-assisted range of motion (AAROM). No swimming strokes.

3. Phase III (Weeks 8 to 11):

    a. Goal: Gradual progression of range of motion exercises. Emphasize good shoulder mechanics when progression through ROM exercises

    b. Progression of PROM, to AAROM, to AROM to normalize ROM

    c. Initiate posterior capsule stretching, cross body adduction stretching as needed

    d. No rotator cuff strengthening exercises. May do scapular, back, and biceps strengthening with light resistance.

4. Phase IV (Weeks 12 and beyond):

    a. Goal: Slow and gradual pain-free progression of ROM and strength in order to return to all normal activities of daily living (ADLs), work, and recreational activities

    b. Gradual increasing stress to the shoulder while returning to normal activities of daily living, work, and recreational activities

    c. If full ROM before 5 months, may discontinue from therapy to return at 5 months for strengthening

    d. Dynamic stabilization exercises and closed chain activity progression

    e. Initially performed in a position of comfort with low stress to the surgical repair in the plane of the scapula (band or light weights)

    f. Rehabilitation activities should be pain free and performed without substitutions or altered movement patterns.

References

1. Strauss E, Frank D, Kubiak E, Kummer F, Rokito A. The effect of the angle of suture anchor insertion on fixation failure at the tendon-suture interface after rotator cuff repair: deadman's angle revisited. Arthroscopy 2009;25(6):597–602

2. Kim YK, Moon SH, Cho SH. Treatment outcomes of single- versus double-row repair for larger than medium-sized rotator cuff tears: the effect of preoperative remnant tendon length. Am J Sports Med 2013;41(10):2270–2277

3. Nicholson GP. Surgical treatment of full-thickness rotator cuff tears. In: Orthopaedic Knowledge Update: Shoulder and Elbow 4. Chapter 15. Amer Academy of Orthopaedic; 2013

4. Lo IK, Burkhart SS. Double-row arthroscopic rotator cuff repair: Re-establishing the footprint of the rotator cuff. Arthroscopy 2003;19(9):1035–1042

5. Virk MS, Bruce B, Hussey KE, et al. Biomechanical performance of medial row suture placement relative to the musculotendinous junction in transosseous equivalent suture bridge double-row rotator cuff repair. Arthroscopy 2017;33(2):242–250

6. Kim DH, Elattrache NS, Tibone JE, et al. Biomechanical comparison of a single-row versus double-row suture anchor technique for rotator cuff repair. Am J Sports Med 2006;34(3):407–414

7. Baums MH, Spahn G, Buchhorn GH, Schultz W, Hofmann L, Klinger HM. Biomechanical and magnetic resonance imaging evaluation of a single- and double-row rotator cuff repair in an in vivo sheep model. Arthroscopy 2012;28(6):769–777

8. Ma CB, Comerford L, Wilson J, Puttlitz CM. Biomechanical evaluation of arthroscopic rotator cuff repairs: double-row compared with single-row fixation. J Bone Joint Surg Am 2006;88(2):403–410

9. Mazzocca AD, Millett PJ, Guanche CA, Santangelo SA, Arciero RA. Arthroscopic single-row versus double-row suture anchor rotator cuff repair. Am J Sports Med 2005;33(12):1861–1868

10. Park MC, ElAttrache NS, Tibone JE, Ahmad CS, Jun BJ, Lee TQ. Part I: Footprint contact characteristics for a transosseous-equivalent rotator cuff repair technique compared with a double-row repair technique. J Shoulder Elbow Surg 2007;16(4):461–468

11. Park MC, Tibone JE, ElAttrache NS, Ahmad CS, Jun BJ, Lee TQ. Part II: Biomechanical assessment for a footprint-restoring transosseous-equivalent rotator cuff repair technique compared with a double-row repair technique. J Shoulder Elbow Surg 2007;16(4):469–476

12. Shi BY, Diaz M, Binkley M, McFarland EG, Srikumaran U. Biomechanical strength of rotator cuff repairs: a systematic review and meta-regression analysis of cadaveric studies. Am J Sports Med 2019;47(8):1984–1993

13. Franceschi F, Ruzzini L, Longo UG, et al. Equivalent clinical results of arthroscopic single-row and double-row suture anchor repair for rotator cuff tears: a randomized controlled trial. Am J Sports Med 2007;35(8):1254–1260

14. Lapner PL, Sabri E, Rakhra K, et al. A multicenter randomized controlled trial comparing single-row with double-row fixation in arthroscopic rotator cuff repair. J Bone Joint Surg Am 2012;94(14):1249–1257

15. Koh KH, Kang KC, Lim TK, Shon MS, Yoo JC. Prospective randomized clinical trial of single- versus double-row suture anchor repair in 2- to 4-cm rotator cuff tears: clinical and magnetic resonance imaging results. Arthroscopy 2011;27(4):453–462

16. Burks RT, Crim J, Brown N, Fink B, Greis PE. A prospective randomized clinical trial comparing arthroscopic single- and double-row rotator cuff repair: magnetic resonance imaging and early clinical evaluation. Am J Sports Med 2009;37(4):674–682

17. Grasso A, Milano G, Salvatore M, Falcone G, Deriu L, Fabbriciani C. Single-row versus double-row arthroscopic rotator cuff repair: a prospective randomized clinical study. Arthroscopy 2009;25(1):4–12

18. Chen M, Xu W, Dong Q, Huang Q, Xie Z, Mao Y. Outcomes of single-row versus double-row arthroscopic rotator cuff repair: a systematic review and meta-analysis of current evidence. Arthroscopy 2013;29(8):1437–1449

19. Millett PJ, Warth RJ, Dornan GJ, Lee JT, Spiegl UJ. Clinical and structural outcomes after arthroscopic single-row versus double-row rotator cuff repair: a systematic review and meta-analysis of level I randomized clinical trials. J Shoulder Elbow Surg 2014;23(4):586–597

20. Sheibani-Rad S, Giveans MR, Arnoczky SP, Bedi A. Arthroscopic single-row versus double-row rotator cuff repair: a meta-analysis of the randomized clinical trials. Arthroscopy 2013;29(2):343–348

21. Carbonel I, Martinez AA, Calvo A, Ripalda J, Herrera A. Single-row versus double-row arthroscopic repair in the treatment of rotator cuff tears: a prospective randomized clinical study. Int Orthop 2012;36(9):1877–1883

22. Park JY, Lhee SH, Choi JH, Park HK, Yu JW, Seo JB. Comparison of the clinical outcomes of single- and double-row repairs in rotator cuff tears. Am J Sports Med 2008;36(7):1310–1316

23. Ma HL, Chiang ER, Wu HT, et al. Clinical outcome and imaging of arthroscopic single-row and double-row rotator cuff repair: a prospective randomized trial. Arthroscopy 2012;28(1):16–24

24. Xu C, Zhao J, Li D. Meta-analysis comparing single-row and double-row repair techniques in the arthroscopic treatment of rotator cuff tears. J Shoulder Elbow Surg 2014;23(2):182–188

25. Ying ZM, Lin T, Yan SG. Arthroscopic single-row versus double-row technique for repairing rotator cuff tears: a systematic review and meta-analysis. Orthop Surg 2014;6(4):300–312

26. Boyer P, Bouthors C, Delcourt T, et al. Arthroscopic double-row cuff repair with suture-bridging: a structural and functional comparison of two techniques. Knee Surg Sports Traumatol Arthrosc 2015;23(2):478–486

27. Park JY, Lhee SH, Oh KS, Moon SG, Hwang JT. Clinical and ultrasonographic outcomes of arthroscopic suture bridge repair for massive rotator cuff tear. Arthroscopy 2013;29(2):280–289

28. McCormick F, Gupta A, Bruce B, et al. Single-row, double-row, and transosseous equivalent techniques for isolated supraspinatus tendon tears with minimal atrophy: A retrospective comparative outcome and radiographic analysis at minimum 2-year followup. Int J Shoulder Surg 2014;8(1):15–20

29. Gerhardt C, Hug K, Pauly S, Marnitz T, Scheibel M. Arthroscopic single-row modified Mason-Allen repair versus double-row suture bridge reconstruction for supraspinatus tendon tears: a matched-pair analysis. Am J Sports Med 2012;40(12):2777–2785

30. Kim KC, Shin HD, Lee WY, Han SC. Repair integrity and functional outcome after arthroscopic rotator cuff repair: double-row versus suture-bridge technique. Am J Sports Med 2012;40(2):294–299

31. Galatz LM, Ball CM, Teefey SA, Middleton WD, Yamaguchi K. The outcome and repair integrity of completely arthroscopically repaired large and massive rotator cuff tears. J Bone Joint Surg Am 2004;86(2):219–224

32. Harryman DT II, Mack LA, Wang KY, Jackins SE, Richardson ML, Matsen FA III. Repairs of the rotator cuff: correlation of functional results with integrity of the cuff. J Bone Joint Surg Am 1991;73(7):982–989

33. Lafosse L, Brozska R, Toussaint B, Gobezie R. The outcome and structural integrity of arthroscopic rotator cuff repair with use of the double-row suture anchor technique. J Bone Joint Surg Am 2007;89(7):1533–1541

34. Boileau P, Brassart N, Watkinson DJ, Carles M, Hatzidakis AM, Krishnan SG. Arthroscopic repair of full-thickness tears of the supraspinatus: does the tendon really heal? J Bone Joint Surg Am 2005;87(6):1229–1240

35. Frank JB, ElAttrache NS, Dines JS, Blackburn A, Crues J, Tibone JE. Repair site integrity after arthroscopic transosseous-equivalent suture-bridge rotator cuff repair. Am J Sports Med 2008;36(8):1496–1503

36. Huijsmans PE, Pritchard MP, Berghs BM, van Rooyen KS, Wallace AL, de Beer JF. Arthroscopic rotator cuff repair with double-row fixation. J Bone Joint Surg Am 2007;89(6):1248–1257

37. Sugaya H, Maeda K, Matsuki K, Moriishi J. Repair integrity and functional outcome after arthroscopic double-row rotator cuff repair: a prospective outcome study. J Bone Joint Surg Am 2007;89(5):953–960

38. Tashjian RZ, Hollins AM, Kim HM, et al. Factors affecting healing rates after arthroscopic double-row rotator cuff repair. Am J Sports Med 2010;38(12):2435-2442

39. Zumstein MA, Jost B, Hempel J, Hodler J, Gerber C. The clinical and structural long-term results of open repair of massive tears of the rotator cuff. J Bone Joint Surg Am 2008;90(11):2423-2431

40. Lee YS, Jeong JY, Park CD, Kang SG, Yoo JC. Evaluation of the risk factors for a rotator cuff retear after repair surgery. Am J Sports Med 2017;45(8):1755-1761

41. Choi CH, Kim SK, Cho MR, et al. Functional outcomes and structural integrity after double-pulley suture bridge rotator cuff repair using serial ultrasonographic examination. J Shoulder Elbow Surg 2012;21(12):1753-1763

42. Liem D, Bartl C, Lichtenberg S, Magosch P, Habermeyer P. Clinical outcome and tendon integrity of arthroscopic versus mini-open supraspinatus tendon repair: a magnetic resonance imaging-controlled matched-pair analysis. Arthroscopy 2007;23(5):514-521

43. Yoo JC, Ahn JH, Koh KH, Lim KS. Rotator cuff integrity after arthroscopic repair for large tears with less-than-optimal footprint coverage. Arthroscopy 2009;25(10):1093-1100

44. Kim JR, Cho YS, Ryu KJ, Kim JH. Clinical and radiographic outcomes after arthroscopic repair of massive rotator cuff tears using a suture bridge technique: assessment of repair integrity on magnetic resonance imaging. Am J Sports Med 2012;40(4):786-793

45. Park JY, Siti HT, Keum JS, Moon SG, Oh KS. Does an arthroscopic suture bridge technique maintain repair integrity? a serial evaluation by ultrasonography. Clin Orthop Relat Res 2010;468(6):1578-1587

46. Sethi PM, Noonan BC, Cunningham J, Shreck E, Miller S. Repair results of 2-tendon rotator cuff tears utilizing the transosseous equivalent technique. J Shoulder Elbow Surg 2010;19(8):1210-1217

47. Hantes ME, Ono Y, Raoulis VA, et al. Arthroscopic single-row versus double-row suture bridge technique for rotator cuff tears in patients younger than 55 years: a prospective comparative study. Am J Sports Med 2018;46(1):116-121

48. Liem D, Lichtenberg S, Magosch P, Habermeyer P. Magnetic resonance imaging of arthroscopic supraspinatus tendon repair. J Bone Joint Surg Am 2007;89(8):1770-1776

49. Mihata T, Watanabe C, Fukunishi K, et al. Functional and structural outcomes of single-row versus double-row versus combined double-row and suture-bridge repair for rotator cuff tears. Am J Sports Med 2011;39(10):2091-2098

50. Duquin TR, Buyea C, Bisson LJ. Which method of rotator cuff repair leads to the highest rate of structural healing? A systematic review. Am J Sports Med 2010;38(4):835-841

51. Hein J, Reilly JM, Chae J, Maerz T, Anderson K. Retear rates after arthroscopic single-row, double-row, and suture bridge rotator cuff repair at a minimum of 1 year of imaging follow-up: a systematic review. Arthroscopy 2015;31(11):2274-2281

52. Jeong JY, Park KM, Sundar S, Yoo JC. Clinical and radiologic outcome of arthroscopic rotator cuff repair: single-row versus transosseous equivalent repair. J Shoulder Elbow Surg 2018;27(6):1021-1029

53. Pennington WT, Gibbons DJ, Bartz BA, et al. Comparative analysis of single-row versus double-row repair of rotator cuff tears. Arthroscopy 2010;26(11):1419-1426

54. Gartsman GM, Drake G, Edwards TB, et al. Ultrasound evaluation of arthroscopic full-thickness supraspinatus rotator cuff repair: single-row versus double-row suture bridge (transosseous equivalent) fixation. Results of a prospective, randomized study. J Shoulder Elbow Surg 2013;22(11):1480-1487

55. Cho NS, Yi JW, Lee BG, Rhee YG. Retear patterns after arthroscopic rotator cuff repair: single-row versus suture bridge technique. Am J Sports Med 2010;38(4):664-671

56. Cho NS, Lee BG, Rhee YG. Arthroscopic rotator cuff repair using a suture bridge technique: is the repair integrity actually maintained? Am J Sports Med 2011;39(10):2108-2116

57. Trantalis JN, Boorman RS, Pletsch K, Lo IK. Medial rotator cuff failure after arthroscopic double-row rotator cuff repair. Arthroscopy 2008;24(6):727-731

58. Christoforetti JJ, Krupp RJ, Singleton SB, Kissenberth MJ, Cook C, Hawkins RJ. Arthroscopic suture bridge transosseus equivalent fixation of rotator cuff tendon preserves intratendinous blood flow at the time of initial fixation. J Shoulder Elbow Surg 2012;21(4):523-530

59. Kim SH, Kim J, Choi YE, Lee HR. Healing disturbance with suture bridge configuration repair in rabbit rotator cuff tear. J Shoulder Elbow Surg 2016;25(3):478-486

60. Urita A, Funakoshi T, Horie T, Nishida M, Iwasaki N. Difference in vascular patterns between transosseous-equivalent and transosseous rotator cuff repair. J Shoulder Elbow Surg 2017;26(1):149-156

61. Rhee YG, Cho NS, Parke CS. Arthroscopic rotator cuff repair using modified Mason-Allen medial row stitch: knotless versus knot-tying suture bridge technique. Am J Sports Med 2012;40(11):2440-2447

62. Tanaka M, Hayashida K, Kobayashi A, Kakiuchi M. Arthroscopic rotator cuff repair with absorbable sutures in the medial-row anchors. Arthroscopy 2015;31(11):2099–2105

63. Kilcoyne KG, Guillaume SG, Hannan CV, Langdale ER, Belkoff SM, Srikumaran U. Anchored transosseous-equivalent versus anchorless transosseous rotator cuff repair: a biomechanical analysis in a cadaveric model. Am J Sports Med 2017;45(10):2364–2371

64. Lee J, Shukla D, Sanchez-Sotelo J. Subscapularis Tears: hidden and forgotten no more. JSES Open access 2018:74–83

65. Denard PJ, Burkhart SS. Arthroscopic Recognition and Repair of the Torn Subscapularis Tendon. Arthroscopy Techniques 2013:e373–e379

66. Thigpen et al. The American Society of Shoulder and Elbow Therapists' consensus statement on rehabilitation following arthroscopic rotator cuff repair. J Shoulder Elbow Surg. 2016 Apr;25(4):521–35

10 Rotator Cuff Reconstruction

Ankit Bansal and Uma Srikumaran

Summary

Prolonged rotator cuff failure, persistent pain and dysfunction, may necessitate reconstructive operations. This chapter outlines various surgical options available for treatment of massive rotator cuff tears. If reparable, then primary tissue healing to bone is ideal. However, if not amenable to repair, then tendon augmentation, reconstruction, or tendon transfers offer reasonable alternatives to reverse shoulder arthroplasty.

Keywords: Massive rotator cuff tears, irreparable, augmentation, reconstruction, tendon-transfer

I. Overview

A. Functional improvement is better if the repaired tendon heals to bone

B. Lower overhead strength reported if rotator cuff (RTC) tendon retears, even though pain level and functional scores remain favorable

C. Biologic augmentation options have been described:

    1. Allograft

    2. Extracellular matrices (ECMs)

    3. Platelet-rich plasma (PRP)

    4. Growth factors

    5. Stem cells

    6. Gene therapy.

D. Risk factors for failure:

    1. Size of tear

    2. Degree of fatty infiltration, muscle atrophy

    3. Patient's age

    4. Prolonged tear chronicity

    5. Fixed or dynamic anterosuperior humeral escape.

II. Relative indications

A. Indicated when diminished potential for tendon healing is suspected

B. Controversial

C. Massive RTC tear >5 cm, or involving more than two tendons

D. Revision surgery for failed previous repair.

III. Contraindications

A. Active infection

B. Substantial glenohumeral arthritis.

IV. Reconstructive options for massive RTC tears

A. Partial repair, margin convergence

B. Primary repair with biologic augmentation

C. Primary repair with structural augmentation

D. RTC reconstruction with structural bridge repair:

1. Allograft, xenograft, nanofiber technology.

E. Superior capsular reconstruction

F. Tendon transfers:

1. Latissimus dorsi

2. Pectoralis major.

V. Partial repair with margin convergence

A. Side-to-side closure of massive, U-shaped RTC tear

B. Combine this with end-on tendon-to-bone repair of the free tendon edge

C. U-shaped tears begin as L-shaped tear, but assume a U shape due to elasticity of the muscle-tendon unit

D. Margin convergence of two-thirds of U-shaped tear reduces free edge strain to one-sixth of initial strain

E. Partial repair of at least half of the infraspinatus is the goal, if complete tendon coverage is not possible.

VI. Biologic augmentation options

A. PRP—Derived from platelets:

1. Randomized prospective double-blind controlled study did not find significant differences in clinical outcomes on magnetic resonance imaging (MRI) with use of PRP

2. Randomized study with autologous platelet-rich fibrin matrix did not yield substantial differences in tendon healing.

B. Mesenchymal stem cells (MSCs):

1. Showed favorable tendon enthesis healing in rat model using anterior cruciate ligament and flexor hallucis longus tendon

2. No clear evidence supporting use of RTC tears:

    a. Unclear whether molecular or cellular signals for appropriate differentiation are present.

C. Growth factors:

1. Fibroblast growth factors (FGF)
2. Cartilage oligomatrix protein (COMP)
3. Platelet-derived growth factor (PDGF)
4. Transforming growth factor beta-1 (TGF-B1)
5. Bone morphogenic proteins 12,13, and 14
6. Further research required to yield appropriate use and indications.

VII. Extracellular matrix augmentation

A. Available as allograft, xenograft, and synthetic ECMs

B. Manufacturing involves physical, chemical, and enzymatic decellularization

C. Can be used as patch to augment primary RTC repair (▶ **Fig. 10.1**):

1. Effective scaffold for aligned cellular growth and collagen assembly
2. Randomized study showed improved tendon healing for two-tendon tears greater than 3 cm.

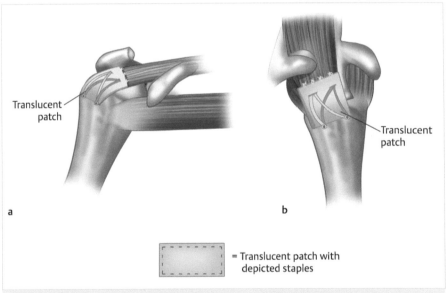

Fig. 10.1 Extracellular matrix augmentation of rotator cuff (RTC) repair: **(a)** coronal view and **(b)** sagittal view.

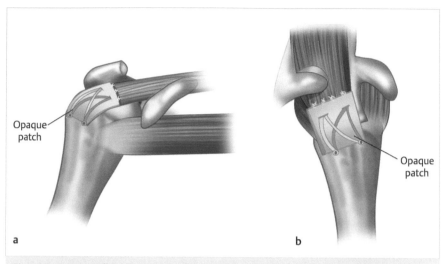

Fig. 10.2 Rotator cuff (RTC) reconstruction with allograft bridge augmentation: **(a)** coronal view and **(b)** sagittal view.

D. Can be used as graft to reconstruct RTC defect, that is, bridge repair (▶ Fig. 10.2):
   1. Serves as tissue bridge between shortened tendon and bone
   2. Level IV series support improved functional outcomes at minimum 2-year follow-up.
E. Xenograft:
   1. Demonstrated no improvement in patient outcomes
   2. 20% of patients had inflammatory response
   3. Decreased postrepair strength, increased shoulder impingement, slower pain resolution, and no decrease in retear rate.
F. Human dermal allograft:
   1. Specific manufacturers have been shown to have improved higher load-to-failure in cadaveric studies
   2. Failure rate in massive RTC tears is reported to be 19%
   3. Histologically, collagen was well-aligned and showed little blood vessel ingrowth
   4. Disadvantages:
      a. Potential for allogenic inflammatory response
      b. Less elastic than autogenic tendon and may contribute to increased retear rates.

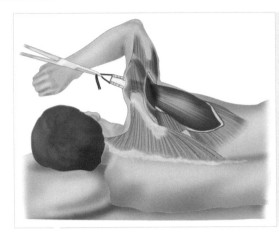

Fig. 10.3 Latissimus tendon transfer to superolateral humeral head.

VIII. Tendon transfers

A. Latissimus dorsi transfer (▶ **Fig. 10.3**):

1. Provides large, vascularized tendon to close the RTC defect in the superolateral humeral head

2. Becomes a humeral head depressor and shoulder external rotator

3. Shown to improve by approximately 20 degrees of flexion, and approximately 7 degrees of external rotation

4. Patients have noted improved extremity strength

5. Can be harvested with humeral insertional bone attachment in an effort to achieve bone-to-bone healing at the greater tuberosity

6. Predictors of a poor outcome following transfer:

   a. Presence of insufficient subscapularis

   b. Pseudoparalysis

   c. Performed as revision operation following previously failed RTC repair

   d. Concomitant unresolved shoulder pathology.

B. Lower trapezius transfer with Achilles allograft elongation (▶ **Fig. 10.4**):

1. Lower trapezius retracts and externally rotates scapula, and inserts on scapular spine

2. Near identical line of pull to infraspinatus muscle

3. Synergistic muscle transfer for posterosuperior RTC tears

4. Has limited excursion compared to latissimus muscle, so needs to be combined with Achilles allograft for elongation

5. Can be performed as open or arthroscopically assisted

6. Has been shown to improve pain, clinical function, and active range of motion in the setting of massive irreparable RTC tears.

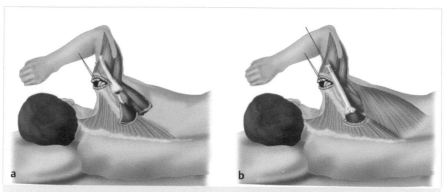

Fig. 10.4 (a, b) Lower trapezius tendon transfer with Achilles allograft elongation.

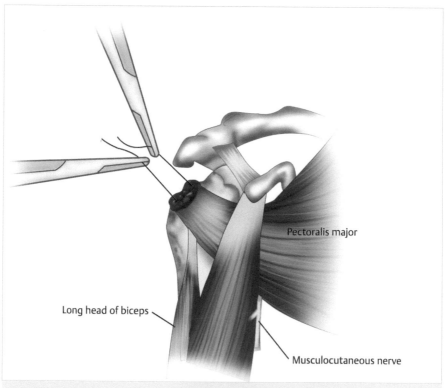

Pectoralis major

Long head of biceps

Musculocutaneous nerve

Fig. 10.5 Pectoralis muscle transfer for subscapularis insufficiency.

C. Pectoralis major transfer (▶ **Fig. 10.5**):

1. Indicated for chronic irreparable subscapularis tears and for anterior glenohumeral instability

2. Presence of lift-off test, lift-off lag, and bear hug test

3. Superior two-thirds of pectoralis major tendon is transferred to the lesser tuberosity at site of subscapularis insertion

4. The sternal head can be transferred, tunneled deep to the clavicular head, such that the clavicular head acts as a fulcrum to more closely mimic subscapularis force vector

5. Nonetheless, force vector remains anterior to the chest wall, whereas the subscapularis is posterior to the chest wall

6. Poor success with transfer in the setting of anterior instability following total shoulder arthroplasty.

Suggested Readings

Cheung EV, Silverio L, Sperling JW. Strategies in biologic augmentation of rotator cuff repair: a review. Clin Orthop Relat Res 2010;468(6):1476–1484

Steinhaus ME, Makhni EC, Cole BJ, Romeo AA, Verma NN. Outcomes after patch use in rotator cuff repair. Arthroscopy 2016;32(8):1676–1690

Thangarajah T, Pendegrass CJ, Shahbazi S, Lambert S, Alexander S, Blunn GW. Augmentation of rotator cuff repair with soft tissue scaffolds. Orthop J Sports Med 2015;3(6):2325967115587495

11 Frozen Shoulder

Matthew Baker and Uma Srikumaran

Summary

Initially described by Duplay as "peri-arthritis" in 1872, Codman coined the term "frozen shoulder" in 1934. He described a condition in which there was insidious onset of shoulder pain associated with stiffness and difficulty in sleeping on the side. He also identified the hallmark of the disease, that is, loss of external rotation and elevation. Naviesar coined the term "adhesive capsulitis" in 1945.

Keywords: Frozen shoulder, adhesive capsuliits

I. Introduction

A. Idiopathic loss of range of motion of the glenohumeral (GH) joint

B. Contracture of the GH joint, scarring of the capsule, and ligamentous complex

C. Histologic evaluation shows capsular fibroblastic proliferation

D. Natural history is that of eventual recovery:

    1. Up to 50% of patients have some residual stiffness/pain.

II. Risk factors

A. Associated with endocrine disorders:

    1. Diabetes mellitus:

        a. Have worse outcomes.

    2. Hyper- or hypothyroid

    3. Other autoimmune disorders.

B. Recent surgery:

    1. Rotator cuff (RTC) repair

    2. Fracture

    3. Breast cancer surgery.

C. Cerebrovascular accident or stroke

D. Parkinson's disease

E. Cardiac disease

F. Prolong immobilization

G. Age 40–60 years

H. Female > Male.

III. Stages

A. Freezing:

    1. Increasing pain and decreased motion

    2. Can last from 6 weeks to 9 months.

B. Frozen:

    1. Pain improves, but motion loss

    2. Can last 4–6 months.

C. Thawing:

    1. Improvement in motion and function

    2. Can take 6–24 months.

IV. Anatomy

A. Coracohumeral ligament and rotator interval have been described as the essential lesion

B. Rotator interval (▶ **Fig. 11.1**):

    1. Triangular region between the anterior border of the supraspinatus and the superior border of the subscapularis

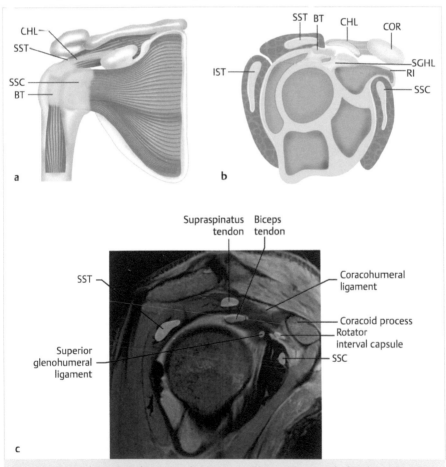

Fig. 11.1 (a–c) Schematic and MRI scan demonstrating the rotator interval, glenohumeral ligaments, and rotator cuff tendons. BT, biceps tendon; CHL, coracohumeral ligament; COR, coracoid process; IST, infraspinatus tendon; RI, rotator interval; SGHL, superior glenohumeral ligament; SST, supraspinatus tendon; SSC , subscapularis.

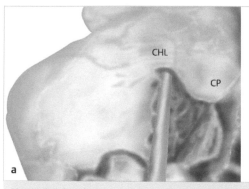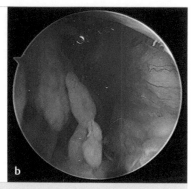

Fig. 11.2 (a) Probe is under the coracohumeral ligament. (b) Arthroscopic view of anterior glenohumeral capsule from posterior portal demonstrating significant synovitis in the rotator cuff interval. The subscapularis tendon is seen running horizontally across the bottom half of the image. CP, coracoid process; CHL, coracohumeral ligament.

    2. Superior glenohumeral ligament (SGHL) and coracohumeral ligament (CHL) (▶ **Fig. 11.2**)

    3. Arthroscopic image of synovitis in frozen shoulder.

V. Presentation/Physical examination

A. Painful loss of motion, especially external rotation

B. Document active and passive range of motion (ROM) in all planes

    1. Loss of both active and passive ROM.

VI. Imaging

A. X-ray can show disuse osteopenia:

    1. Look for evidence of previous surgery, fracture, arthritis, or calcific tendonitis.

B. Magnetic resonance imaging (MRI):

    1. With arthrogram, loss of the axillary recess → capsular contracture.

VII. Treatment

A. Nonoperative:

    1. Nonsteroidal anti-inflammatory drugs (NSAIDs), oral steroids, GH steroid injections, physical therapy, and saline joint distention

    2. Therapy should focus on pain-free stretching.

B. Operative:

    1. Manipulation under anesthesia (MUA):

        a. Risk of fracture.

2. Arthroscopic capsular release (ACR):
   a. 180 degrees versus 270 degrees versus 360 degrees release:
      i. Risk of injury to the axillary nerve with complete release
      ii. Improved immediate ROM with increased release and can avoid manipulation with complete release (360 degrees).
   b. Important to release CHL.
3. Indicated after failure of nonoperative measures.

VIII. Results

A. Most of the time (90%), function and ROM return to normal—can take up to 3 years
B. Significant improvement in ROM and pain scores after MUA and ACR
C. Early intervention tends to improve the outcome
   1. 80–90% patient satisfaction with MUA and ACR.
D. Typically does not recur in the same shoulder but can present on the contralateral side.

Suggested Readings

Ahmad D, Hashim JA, Asim HM. Outcome of manipulation under anaesthesia in adhesive capsulitis patients. J Coll Physicians Surg Pak 2014;24(4):293–294

Brealey S, Armstrong AL, Brooksbank A, et al. United Kingdom Frozen Shoulder Trial (UK FROST), multi-centre, randomised, 12 month, parallel group, superiority study to compare the clinical and cost-effectiveness of early structured physiotherapy versus manipulation under anaesthesia versus arthroscopic capsular release for patients referred to secondary care with a primary frozen shoulder: study protocol for a randomised controlled trial. Trials 2017;18(1):614 10.1186/s13063-017-2352-2

Burkart AC, Debski RE. Anatomy and function of the glenohumeral ligaments in anterior shoulder instability. Clin Orthop Relat Res 2002; (400):32–39

Cinar M, Akpinar S, Derincek A, Circi E, Uysal M. Comparison of arthroscopic capsular release in diabetic and idiopathic frozen shoulder patients. Arch Orthop Trauma Surg 2010;130(3):401–406

Cvetanovich GL, Leroux T, Hamamoto JT, Higgins JD, Romeo AA, Verma NN. Arthroscopic 360° capsular release for adhesive capsulitis in the lateral decubitus position. Arthrosc Tech 2016;5(5):e1033–e1038. doi:10.1016/j.eats.2016.05.007

Dias R, Cutts S, Massoud S. Frozen shoulder. BMJ 2005;331(7530):1453–1456

Flannery O, Mullett H, Colville J. Adhesive shoulder capsulitis: does the timing of manipulation influence outcome? Acta Orthop Belg 2007;73(1):21–25

Hagiwara Y, Ando A, Kanazawa K, et al. Arthroscopic coracohumeral ligament release for patients with frozen shoulder. Arthrosc Tech 2017;7(1):e1–e5

Hwang KR, Murrell GA, Millar NL, Bonar F, Lam P, Walton JR. Advanced glycation end products in idiopathic frozen shoulders. J Shoulder Elbow Surg 2016;25(6):981–988

Maund E, Craig D, Suekarran S, et al. Management of frozen shoulder: a systematic review and cost-effectiveness analysis. Health Technol Assess 2012;16(11):1–264

Musil D, Sadovský P, Stehlík J, Filip L, Vodicka Z. [Arthroscopic capsular release in frozen shoulder syndrome]. Acta Chir Orthop Traumatol Cech 2009;76(2):98–103

Neviaser AS, Neviaser RJ. Adhesive capsulitis of the shoulder. J Am Acad Orthop Surg 2011;19(9):536–542

Page MJ, Green S, Kramer S, et al. Manual therapy and exercise for adhesive capsulitis (frozen shoulder). Cochrane Database Syst Rev 2014; (8):CD011275

Page MJ, Green S, Kramer S, Johnston RV, McBain B, Buchbinder R. Electrotherapy modalities for adhesive capsulitis (frozen shoulder). Cochrane Database Syst Rev 2014; (10):CD011324

Shaffer B, Tibone JE, Kerlan RK. Frozen shoulder: a long-term follow-up. J Bone Joint Surg Am 1992;74(5):738–746

Sheridan MA, Hannafin JA. Upper extremity: emphasis on frozen shoulder. Orthop Clin North Am 2006;37(4):531–539

Tasto JP, Elias DW. Adhesive capsulitis. Sports Med Arthrosc Rev 2007;15(4):216–221

12 Anterior Shoulder Instability

Alexander E. Loeb and Uma Srikumaran

Summary

An anterior shoulder dislocation commonly presents as an acute shoulder injury from direct trauma. Young, active males and patients with glenoid bone loss are at highest risk of recurrent dislocation. First-time dislocators without significant risk factors can be managed with reduction, immobilization, and physical therapy, while high-risk patients and recurrent dislocators may be treated with surgery.

Keywords: Anterior shoulder dislocation, anterior shoulder instability

I. General overview

A. Laxity: Physiologic translation of the humeral head on glenoid

B. Instability: Pathologic translation of the humeral head on the glenoid causing pain or dysfunction

C. Anteroinferior stability most common

D. Static and dynamic stabilizers responsible for stability.

II. Anatomy (►Fig. 12.1)

A. Glenohumeral joint resembles a ball on tee:
    1. Articulating surface of humeral head is 3× larger than the surface of the glenoid.

B. Glenoid:
    1. Glenoid is pear-shaped, broader inferiorly than superiorly
    2. Provides 50% of the depth of the glenohumeral joint:
        a. Labrum provides the other 50% of depth.
    3. Slightly concave:
        a. Cartilage thicker at the periphery, bare spot centrally.
    4. Retroversion and inclination varies widely, approximately 0–5 degrees retroverted, 5 degrees inclined.

C. Humerus:
    1. Greater and lesser tuberosities are sites of rotator cuff insertion
    2. Retroverted 30 degrees from the transepicondylar axis, 130 degrees neck–shaft angle.

D. Labrum:
    1. Provides 50% of the depth of glenohumeral joint
    2. Increases glenohumeral contact
    3. Provides conforming seal:
        a. Negative intra-articular pressure.

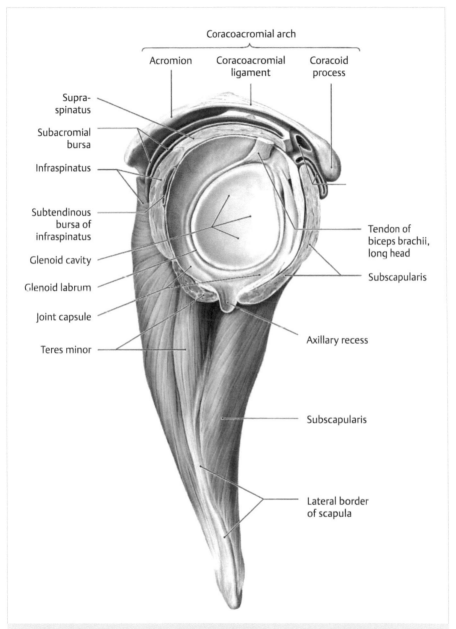

Fig. 12.1 Shoulder anatomy. (Source: Schuenke M, Schulte E. General Anatomy and the Musculoskeletal System: Thieme Atlas of Anatomy. New York: Thieme; 2005. Illustration by Karl Wesker.)

E. Ligaments:
1. Inferior glenohumeral ligament:
    a. Anterior band is primary restraint to anterior translation with the shoulder in 90 degrees abduction and external rotation.
2. Superior glenohumeral ligament:
    a. Primary restraint to inferior translation with the arm in adduction.
3. Middle glenohumeral ligament:
    a. Primary restraint to anterior translation with the arm in adduction as well as 45 degrees abduction and external rotation.

F. Musculature:
1. Provide dynamic stabilization by compression into the glenoid concavity:
    a. Rotator cuff provides dynamic stabilization against anteroinferior translation:
        i.   Supraspinatus
        ii. Infraspinatus
        iii. Teres minor
        iv. Subscapularis.
    b. Other contributors: Teres major, latissimus dorsi, long head of biceps brachii, pectoralis major, and deltoid.

III. Pathogenesis

A. Instability can be traumatic, acquired, or atraumatic:
1. Trauma involves direct impact or anterior directed force with the arm abducted and externally rotated:
    a. Typically young, athletic population
    b. Male to female ratio in this population is 9:1.
2. Acquired instability through multiple microtrauma events, for example, in overhead athletes
3. Atraumatic, typically involves congenital anatomic deformities, connective tissue disorders, and multidirectional instability.

B. Bankart lesion:
1. Detachment of the anteroinferior labrum from the glenoid at its inferior glenohumeral ligament attachment
2. Pathognomonic for anteroinferior instability
3. Present in 90% of glenohumeral dislocations.

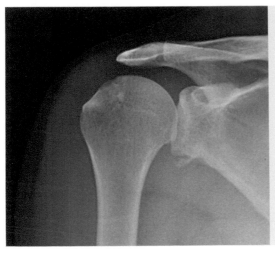

Fig. 12.2 Anteroposterior radiograph with bony Bankart lesion.

C. Bony Bankart lesion (▶Fig. 12.2):
  1. Anteroinferior glenoid avulsion/shear fracture in association with above findings
  2. Present in half of recurrent dislocators
  3. Should be addressed at time of surgery or will remain at risk for instability
  4. Bony defect >20% is highly unstable, requires fixation/Bristow/Latarjet.

D. Humeral avulsion of glenohumeral ligament (HAGL) lesion:
  1. Results from avulsion of inferior glenohumeral ligament from its insertion on the humerus.

E. Glenoid labral articular defect (GLAD) lesion:
  1. Articular cartilage sheared off with labrum.

F. Anterior labroligamentous periosteal sleeve avulsion (ALPSA) lesion (▶Fig. 12.3):
  1. Labrum is avulsed with anterior glenoid neck periosteum
  2. At risk for scarring down more medially, resulting in recurrent instability.

G. Hill-Sachs lesion (▶Fig. 12.4):
  1. Impaction fracture in the posterosuperior humeral head
  2. Head impaction results from contact with glenoid rim
  3. Pathognomonic for anterior dislocation
  4. Present in 80% of traumatic dislocations
  5. May engage the glenoid and cause catching, recurrent dislocation or subluxation, or irreducibility.

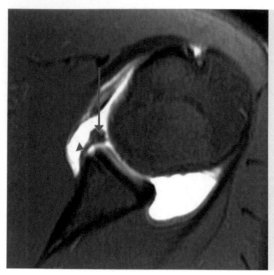

Fig. 12.3 Magnetic resonance imaging (MRI) arthrogram of anterior labroligamentous periosteal sleeve avulsion (ALPSA) lesion.

H. Laxity:

1. Recurrent subluxations and dislocations lead to attenuation and lengthening of the middle and inferior glenohumeral ligaments

2. Less static stabilization results in more instability events, a vicious cycle

3. Teenagers have 90% chance of recurrent dislocation.

I. Other injuries:

1. Greater tuberosity fractures associated with dislocations in the elderly

2. Axillary nerve transient neurapraxia in 5% of traumatic dislocations

3. Rotator cuff tears in 30% of patients younger than 40 years, more common in elderly.

IV. Imaging

A. Radiographs:

1. Grashey (true anteroposterior [AP]):

   a. Taken perpendicular to the plane of the scapula.

2. AP with internal rotation:

   a. May demonstrate Hill-Sachs lesion.

3. Scapular Y:

   a. Taken in the plane of the scapula

   b. Glenohumeral reduction may be difficult to assess.

4. Axillary:

   a. Better orthogonal assessment of glenohumeral reduction.

5. Other views include Velpeau (alternative axillary), West Point axillary (good view of anteroinferior glenoid rim), and Stryker notch (evaluate for Hill-Sachs lesion).

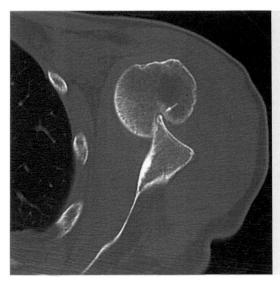

Fig. 12.4 Computed tomography (CT) image with engaging Hill-Sachs lesion.

B. Computed tomography (CT):
    1. Warranted for further workup and preoperative evaluation of glenoid fractures
    2. Indicated for revision evaluation, instability or apprehension at low degrees of abduction or low-energy instability, and significant laxity
    3. Three-dimensional reconstructions help to quantify bone loss.

C. Magnetic resonance imaging (MRI):
    1. With intra-articular contrast (arthrogram), increases sensitivity for detection of labral, rotator cuff, and cartilage pathology
    2. Best for evaluating soft tissue and labral injury
    3. May demonstrate bony lesions not seen on radiograph.

V. Evaluation

A. History:
    1. Important to elicit history of prior instability events/trauma:
        a. Arm position at time of instability
        b. Number of formal reductions
        c. Amount of force needed for most recent dislocation versus first dislocation.
    2. Feelings of instability may represent laxity or subluxation
    3. Provocative maneuvers that produce pain
    4. Pain in a younger patient or with abnormal motion.

B. Physical examination:
    1. Muscle atrophy and strength examination for all shoulder girdle muscles
    2. Range of motion, passive and active
    3. Contralateral shoulder comparison

4. Load and shift:
   a. In 45 degrees of abduction, load the glenohumeral joint with axial load and shift the humeral head anteriorly
   b. Grade 0: Normal glenohumeral translation
   c. 1+: Translation to the glenoid rim but not over
   d. 2+: Translation over the glenoid rim but spontaneously reduces
   e. 3+: Translation over the glenoid rim, remains locked anteriorly until manually reduced.
5. Sulcus test:
   a. Inferior traction force on adducted arm, sulcus forms at superior humeral head
   b. 1+: <1 cm acromiohumeral interval
   c. 2+: 1–2 cm acromiohumeral interval
   d. 3+: >2 cm acromiohumeral interval
   e. External rotation should eliminate sulcus sign; if not, consider rotator interval deficiency.
6. Anterior apprehension:
   a. Supine, arm in 90 degrees abduction and external rotation, slight anterior force on humeral head
   b. Patient experiences sensation of instability
   c. May experience instability without any anterior force.
7. Anterior relocation:
   a. After apprehension test is performed, with arm still in abduction and external rotation, a posterior directed force applied to the humeral head
   b. Patient experiences sensation of return of stability
   c. Can be performed before apprehension test; once posterior force is removed, a sense of instability is positive for apprehension.
8. Shoulder-specific hyperlaxity:
   a. A 2+ load and shift test in two planes (anterior, posterior, inferior)
   b. With arm at side, hyperexternal rotation to >85 degrees
   c. With shoulder in neutral rotation, abduction >120 degrees
   d. Above findings may indicate multidirectional instability.
9. Generalized hyperlaxity:
   a. Beighton score: Positive for hyperlaxity if ≥5/9 points in adults, ≥6/9 in children:
      i. Small finger metacarpophalangeal joint extension beyond 90 degrees (1 point for each side)
      ii. Thumb can touch forearm with passive wrist flexion (1 point for each side)
      iii. Elbow hyperextension greater than 10 degrees (1 point for each side)

    iv. Knee hyperextension greater than 10 degrees (1 point for each side)

    v. Bending from the waist with knees straight, hands can lie flat on the floor (1 point).

VI. Treatment

A. Acute dislocation:
1. Reduction techniques:
   a. Pain control and muscle relaxation is critical:
      i. Consider intra-articular lidocaine or sedation
      ii. Risk of fracture or further soft tissue damage if not relaxed.
   b. Traction-countertraction
   c. Gradual manipulation into abduction and external rotation may disengage Hill-Sachs lesion
   d. Stimson gravity technique
   e. Scapular manipulation.
2. Sling immobilization followed by physical therapy
3. Risk factors for recurrence:
   a. Age <20 years old (*~80–90% recurrence*)
   b. Male
   c. Contact sports
   d. Hyperlaxity
   e. Glenoid bone loss >20% ("inverted pear" glenoid).
4. Should consider operative intervention on patients with abovementioned risk factors.

B. Nonoperative management:
1. Physical therapy for range of motion, scapular stabilization/strengthening, rotator cuff strengthening, and proprioception.

C. Operative intervention:
1. Examination under anesthesia
   a. Confirm with clinical physical examination
   b. Compare to contralateral shoulder.
2. Arthroscopic Bankart repair (▶ **Fig. 12.5**):
   a. Indicated for recurrent instability or first-time dislocators with abovementioned risk factors
   b. Capsular plication at the time of labral repair
   c. Use three or more anchors to reduce risk of failure
   d. Anchors typically placed from 2 o'clock to 6 o'clock position for anteroinferior Bankart defect.

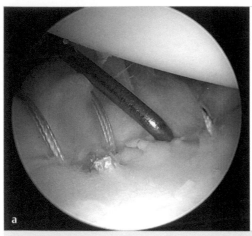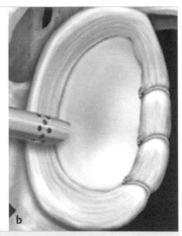

Fig. 12.5 (a, b) Illustration and intraoperative arthroscopic view of arthroscopic labral repair.

3. Open Bankart repair:
   a. Indicated for >20% glenoid bone loss requiring open reduction internal fixation.
4. Remplissage:
   a. Posterior capsulodesis/infraspinatus tenodesis used to augment above repairs in patients with an engaging Hill-Sachs lesion
   b. May result in some loss of external rotation.
5. Bony procedures:
   a. Bone grafting of Hill-Sachs lesion considered for defects >40% of articular surface
   b. Latarjet or Bristow coracoid transfers:
      i. Indicated for glenoid bone loss or recurrent anterior instability with failed Bankart repair
      ii. Iliac crest cortica l bone graft can be used in revision setting.
6. Operative treatment of contact and overhead athletes, but controversial in hyperlax patients.

VII. Complications

A. Recurrence:
   1. Unrecognized glenoid bone loss
   2. Fewer than three suture anchors
   3. Overall recurrence rate of about 10–15% with arthroscopic surgery

4. More than 70% risk of failure of arthroscopic surgery if three or more of the following are present:

   a. Teenage male

   b. Contact athlete

   c. Shoulder hyperlaxity

   d. Hill-Sachs lesion on external rotation AP radiograph

   e. Loss of glenoid contour on radiograph.

5. Medical comorbidities such as seizure disorder should be well controlled with medical therapy before repair is attempted.

B. Stiffness:

   1. Higher incidence after open procedures

   2. Typically associated with coracoid transfer procedures and remplissage.

C. Infection:

   1. Rare in arthroscopy

   2. Cultures should be held for 2 weeks for *Propionibacterium acnes.*

D. Hardware or graft failure.

Suggested Readings

Arciero RA, Wheeler JH, Ryan JB, McBride JT. Arthroscopic Bankart repair versus nonoperative treatment for acute, initial anterior shoulder dislocations. Am J Sports Med 1994;22(5):589–594

Boileau P, Villalba M, Héry JY, Balg F, Ahrens P, Neyton L. Risk factors for recurrence of shoulder instability after arthroscopic Bankart repair. J Bone Joint Surg Am 2006;88(8):1755–1763

Bottoni CR, Smith EL, Berkowitz MJ, Towle RB, Moore JH. Arthroscopic versus open shoulder stabilization for recurrent anterior instability: a prospective randomized clinical trial. Am J Sports Med 2006;34(11):1730–1737

Burkhart SS, De Beer JF. Traumatic glenohumeral bone defects and their relationship to failure of arthroscopic Bankart repairs: significance of the inverted-pear glenoid and the humeral engaging Hill-Sachs lesion. Arthroscopy 2000;16:6776–94

Cameron KL, Mountcastle SB, Nelson BJ, et al. History of shoulder instability and subsequent injury during four years of follow-up: a survival analysis. J Bone Joint Surg Am 2013;95(5):439–445

Hovelius L, Olofsson A, Sandström B, et al. Nonoperative treatment of primary anterior shoulder dislocation in patients forty years of age and younger. a prospective twenty-five-year follow-up. J Bone Joint Surg Am 2008;90(5):945–952

Robinson CM, Jenkins PJ, White TO, Ker A, Will E. Primary arthroscopic stabilization for a first-time anterior dislocation of the shoulder: a randomized, double-blind trial. J Bone Joint Surg Am 2008;90(4):708–721

13 Posterior Shoulder Instability

Alexander E. Loeb and Uma Srikumaran

Summary

A posterior shoulder dislocation can present as an acute shoulder injury, frequently associated with seizures or trauma, and is frequently missed in the Emergency Department. Posterior shoulder instability may present as chronic shoulder pain with the shoulder adducted and flexed as a result of repetitive microtrauma. First-time dislocators are typically managed with reduction, immobilization, and physical therapy, while chronic instability and associated fractures can be managed with surgery.

Keywords: Posterior shoulder instability, posterior shoulder dislocation

I. General overview

A. Laxity: Physiologic translation of the humeral head on glenoid

B. Instability: Pathologic translation of the humeral head on the glenoid causing pain or dysfunction

C. Posterior instability less common than anterior instability: 2–10% of shoulder dislocations

D. However, 50% of posterior shoulder dislocations seen in the Emergency Department are missed on initial evaluation.

II. Anatomy (▶Fig. 13.1)

A. Glenohumeral joint resembles a ball on tee:

    1. Articulating surface of humeral head is 3× larger than the surface of the glenoid.

B. Glenoid:

    1. Glenoid is pear-shaped, broader inferiorly than superiorly

    2. Provides 50% of the depth of the glenohumeral joint:

        a. Labrum provides the other 50% of depth.

    3. Slightly concave:

        a. Cartilage thicker at the periphery, bare spot centrally.

    4. Retroversion and inclination varies widely, approximately 0–5 degrees retroverted, 5 degrees inclined.

C. Humerus:

    1. Greater and lesser tuberosities are sites of rotator cuff insertion

    2. Retroverted 30 degrees from the transepicondylar axis, 130 degrees neck–shaft angle

D. Labrum:

    1. Provides 50% of the depth of glenohumeral joint

    2. Increases glenohumeral contact

    3. Provides conforming seal:

        a. Negative intra-articular pressure.

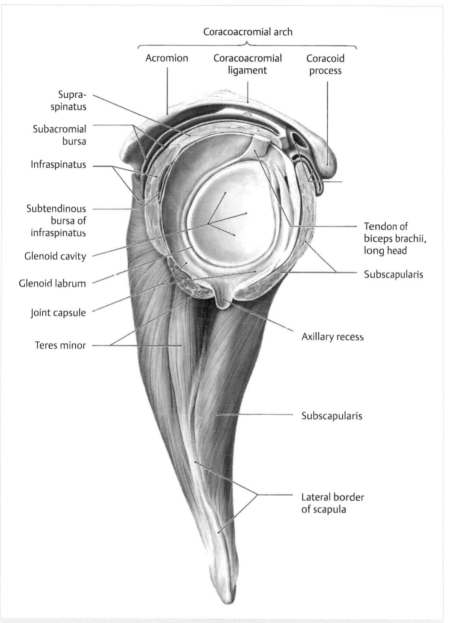

Fig. 13.1 Shoulder anatomy. (Source: Schuenke M, Schulte E. General Anatomy and the Musculoskeletal System: Thieme Atlas of Anatomy. New York: Thieme; 2005. Illustration by Karl Wesker.)

E. Capsule:

    1. Posterior capsule only a few millimeters thick.

F. Ligaments:
1. Inferior glenohumeral ligament:
    a. Posterior band is primary restraint to posterior translation with the shoulder in abduction and internal rotation (pressing activity, follow-through phase of throwing).
2. Superior glenohumeral ligament:
    a. Primary restraint to inferior translation with the arm in adduction.
3. Coracohumeral ligament:
    a. Primary restraint to posterior translation with the arm in forward flexion, adduction, and internal rotation (fall on outstretched hands).
4. Middle glenohumeral ligament:
    a. Secondary restraint to posterior translation with the arm in adduction.
G. Musculature:
1. Provide dynamic stabilization by compression into the glenoid concavity:
    a. Rotator cuff:
        i. Subscapularis:
            • Provides dynamic stabilization against posterior translation
            • Primary restraint to posterior translation in external rotation.
        ii. Supraspinatus
        iii. Infraspinatus
        iv. Teres minor.
    b. Other contributors: Teres major, latissimus dorsi, long head of biceps brachii, pectoralis major, and deltoid.

III. Pathogenesis

A. Posterior instability is generally acute or chronic:
1. Acute etiologies:
    a. Direct trauma:
        i. 50% of cases missed in Emergency Department
        ii. Posterior directed force on the glenohumeral joint.
    b. Seizures or electrocution:
        i. Intense muscle contraction dislocates humeral head
        ii. Anterior dislocations more common with seizures, but proportion of posterior dislocations is higher.
2. Chronic etiologies:
    a. Microtrauma causing posterior capsule attenuation and stretching, leading to instability:
        i. Commonly presents as vague, deep pain with activity, not as frank instability

      ii. At risk activities include impact or load-bearing with the shoulder in a flexed and adducted position

      iii. Commonly seen in weightlifters (bench press), offensive linemen, some overhead athletes, and pitchers.

  3. Glenoid hypoplasia or extreme retroversion as a cause of instability is rare:

    a. Congenital defects such as Erb's palsy may be at risk

    b. May predispose to recurrent instability or labral tears.

B. Posterior Bankart lesion:

  1. Detachment of the posteroinferior labrum from the glenoid at its inferior glenohumeral ligament attachment

  2. Pathognomonic for posteroinferior instability.

C. Posterior Bony Bankart lesion:

  1. Posteroinferior glenoid rim avulsion/shear fracture often in association with above findings.

D. Kim lesion:

  1. Avulsion of the deep posteroinferior labrum as above but with superficial labrum intact to glenoid.

E. Posterior humeral avulsion of glenohumeral ligament (HAGL)

  1. Avulsion of the posterior band of the inferior glenohumeral ligament from the humerus.

F. Posterior labral cyst:

  1. Cyst forms with valve-like effect of synovial fluid passing through labral defect

  2. Commonly seen in chronic posterior instability presentations.

G. Reverse Hill-Sachs lesion (▶ Fig. 13.2):

  1. Impaction fracture in the anterosuperior humeral head

  2. Head impaction results from contact with glenoid rim

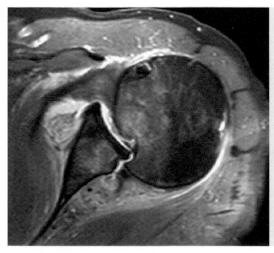

Fig. 13.2 Magnetic resonance imaging (MRI) demonstrating chronic engaging reverse Hill-Sachs lesion.

3. Pathognomonic for posterior dislocation

4. May engage the glenoid and cause catching, recurrent dislocation or subluxation, or irreducibility.

H. Lesser tuberosity fracture:

1. May present with acute/traumatic posterior dislocations.

IV. Imaging

A. Radiographs:

1. Grashey (true anteroposterior [AP]):

   a. Taken perpendicular to the plane of the scapula

   b. Unlikely to demonstrate reverse Hill-Sachs lesion

   c. Lightbulb sign (dislocated humeral head is internally rotated, appears to lose neck–shaft angle, and looks symmetric).

2. Scapular Y:

   a. Taken in the plane of the scapula

   b. Glenohumeral reduction may be difficult to assess.

3. Axillary:

   a. Better orthogonal assessment of glenohumeral reduction

   b. Necessary even in late presentations to rule out chronic dislocation.

4. Other views include Velpeau (alternative axillary), supine West Point axillary (good view of posteroinferior glenoid rim), and reverse Stryker notch (evaluate for reverse Hill-Sachs lesion).

B. Computed tomography (CT):

1. Warranted for further workup and preoperative evaluation of glenoid fractures

2. Indicated for evaluation in a revision setting with persistent posterior instability, apprehension, and laxity

3. Help to quantify bone loss, for example, in chronic dislocations.

C. Magnetic resonance imaging (MRI):

1. Best for posterior labrum and soft tissue evaluation

2. May demonstrate bony lesions not seen on radiograph

3. Indicated for history of posterior pain or instability without acute dislocation.

V. Evaluation

A. History:

1. Elicit history of prior acute/traumatic instability events

2. Provocative maneuvers that produce pain

3. Associated conditions such as seizure disorder

4. At-risk repetitive actions/occupations (weightlifters, offensive linemen, pitchers, and similar actions)

5. Chronic instability typically presents as vague, deep joint pain with flexed, adducted, and internally rotated arm under load

6. Chronic dislocation may present late/may be missed on prior evaluations.

B. Physical examination:

1. Muscle atrophy and strength examination for all shoulder girdle muscles

2. Range of motion, passive and active:

   a. In chronic, missed posterior dislocations, shoulder may be locked in internal rotation; inability to externally rotate is a key finding for chronic dislocation.

3. Contralateral shoulder comparison

4. Posterior load and shift:

   a. In 45 degrees of abduction and 45 degrees of forward flexion, load the glenohumeral joint with axial load and shift the humeral head posteriorly

   b. Grade 0: Normal glenohumeral translation

   c. 1+: Translation to the glenoid rim but not over

   d. 2+: Translation over the glenoid rim but spontaneously reduces

   e. 3+: Translation over the glenoid rim, remains locked posteriorly until manually reduced.

5. Kim test (▶ **Fig. 13.3**):

   a. With arm in 90 degrees of abduction, full internal rotation, with elbow bent

   b. Humerus is loaded axially and arm is adducted into 45 degrees of forward flexion

   c. Other hand provides posteroinferior force on the proximal humerus

   d. Pain is a positive test.

6. Jerk test:

   a. In 90 degrees of abduction, full internal rotation, with elbow bent

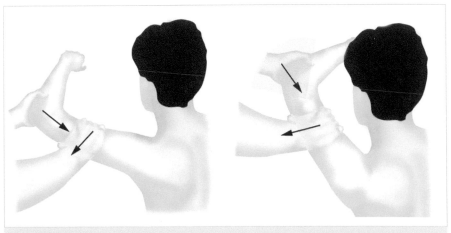

Fig. 13.3 Kim test.

    b. Humerus is loaded axially and arm is adducted into forward flexion

    c. A palpable clunk is positive test

    d. When combined with positive Kim test, 97% sensitive for a posterior labral tear.

7. Posterior stress:

    a. Supine, arm in adduction, 90 degrees forward flexion, internal rotation, with elbow bent

    b. Humerus is loaded axially with a posterior-directed force

    c. Patient experiences pain and sensation of instability.

8. Shoulder-specific hyperlaxity:

    a. A 2+ load and shift test in two planes (anterior, posterior, inferior)

    b. With arm at side, hyperexternal rotation to >85 degrees

    c. With shoulder in neutral rotation, abduction >120 degrees

    d. Above findings may indicate multidirectional instability.

9. Generalized hyperlaxity:

    a. Beighton score: Positive for hyperlaxity if ≥5/9 points in adults, ≥6/9 in children:

        i. Small finger metacarpophalangeal joint extension beyond 90 degrees (1 point for each side)

        ii. Thumb can touch forearm with passive wrist flexion (1 point for each side)

        iii. Elbow hyperextension greater than 10 degrees (1 point for each side)

        iv. Knee hyperextension greater than 10 degrees (1 point for each side)

        v. Bending from the waist with knees straight, hands can lie flat on the floor (1 point).

VI. Treatment

A. Acute dislocation:

  1. Reduction techniques:

    a. Most dislocations reduce spontaneously, and thus are commonly missed

    b. Pain control and muscle relaxation is critical:

        i. Consider intra-articular lidocaine or sedation

        ii. Risk of fracture or further soft tissue damage if not relaxed.

    c. Traction-countertraction

    d. Boss-Holzach-Matter self-assisted technique:

        i. Fingers are interdigitated over ipsilateral knee, patient leans back and lets scapula protract with anterior traction.

B. Nonoperative management:

  1. Shoulder immobilization in 10–20 degrees of external rotation for 6 weeks

  2. Physical therapy with range of motion exercises, scapular stabilizer strengthening, rotator cuff strengthening, and proprioception

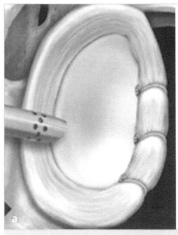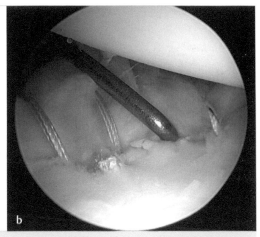

Fig. 13.4 (a, b) Illustration and intraoperative arthroscopic view of an arthroscopic labral repair.

3. Activity modification, avoiding activities with adduction, forward flexion, and internal rotation.

C. Operative intervention:

1. Examination under anesthesia:

   a. Confirm with clinical physical examination

   b. Compare to contralateral shoulder.

2. Arthroscopic posterior labral repair (▶ Fig. 13.4):

   a. Indicated for recurrent posterior shoulder instability or pain with loading in flexion and adduction which fails physical therapy

   b. Posterior capsular shift or plication may be needed if hyperlax

   c. Lateral positioning may afford better posterior labrum exposure

   d. Posterior portal may be slightly lateral to better access the glenoid rim for anchor placement.

3. Open reduction with subscapularis/lesser tuberosity transfer to reverse Hill-Sachs lesion:

   a. Indicated for chronic dislocations and for reverse Hill-Sachs lesions >40% of the articular surface.

4. Hemiarthroplasty or total shoulder arthroplasty:

   a. Consider in chronic dislocations, reverse Hill-Sachs lesions >40% of the articular surface, or with significant humeral head damage or glenohumeral arthritis.

VII. Complications

A. Stiffness:

1. With both long-term nonoperative immobilization and postoperative treatment.

B.   Recurrence:

   1.   0–8% rate of recurrence with arthroscopic surgery.

C.   Arthritis:

   1.   Early development in missed chronic dislocations.

D.   Infection:

   1.   Rare in arthroscopy

   2.   Cultures should be held for 2 weeks for *Propionibacterium acnes.*

E.   Hardware or graft failure

F.   Anterior subluxation:

   1.   If posterior capsule overtightened, it can also lead to coracoid impingement.

Suggested Readings

Bradley JP, McClincy MP, Arner JW, Tejwani SG. Arthroscopic capsulolabral reconstruction for posterior instability of the shoulder: a prospective study of 200 shoulders. Am J Sports Med 2013;41(9):2005–2014

Kim SH, Ha KI, Park JH, et al. Arthroscopic posterior labral repair and capsular shift for traumatic unidirectional recurrent posterior subluxation of the shoulder. J Bone Joint Surg Am 2003;85(8):1479–1487

Kim SH, Park JS, Jeong WK, Shin SK. The Kim test: a novel test for posteroinferior labral lesion of the shoulder—a comparison to the jerk test. Am J Sports Med 2005;33(8):1188–1192

Walch G, Ascani C, Boulahia A, Nové-Josserand L, Edwards TB. Static posterior subluxation of the humeral head: an unrecognized entity responsible for glenohumeral osteoarthritis in the young adult. J Shoulder Elbow Surg 2002;11(4):309–314

14 Shoulder Stabilization Procedures

Eric G. Huish Jr and Uma Srikumaran

Summary

Glenohumeral instability frequently requires surgical intervention to prevent recurrence. Various techniques are utilized depending on the direction of instability and the presence of soft tissue and/or bony lesions. New implants and techniques have made arthroscopic surgery more common.

Keywords: Glenohumeral instability, bankart, latarjet, hill sachs, HAGL

I. Anterior instability

A. Accounts for the majority of glenohumeral dislocations

B. Indications for surgical treatment:

    1. Recurrent instability

    2. First-time dislocation, under 25 years old.

C. Contraindications:

    1. Voluntary dislocators.

D. Associated lesions:

    1. Bankart lesion:

        a. Soft tissue (▶ **Fig. 14.1**)

        b. Bony.

    2. Hill-Sachs lesion (▶ **Fig. 14.1**)

    3. Humeral avulsion of the inferior glenohumeral ligament (HAGL) (▶ **Fig. 14.2**).

E. Procedures for soft tissue lesions:

    1. Bankart repair +/– capsular shift:

        a. Primary treatment of anteroinferior instability with Bankart lesion

        b. Commonly performed with suture anchors

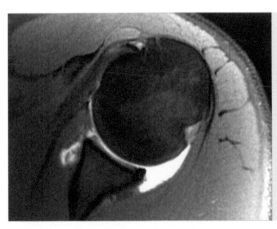

Fig. 14.1 Axial T2 magnetic resonance imaging (MRI) showing Bankart and Hill-Sachs lesions.

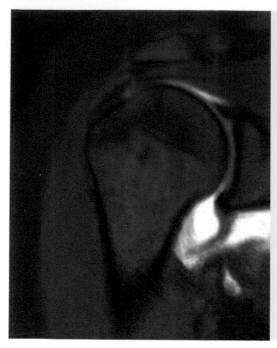

Fig. 14.2 Coronal T2 magnetic resonance imaging (MRI) showing humeral avulsion of the inferior glenohumeral ligament lesion (HAGL).

   c. Can be done arthroscopically or by open procedure:

      i. Similar results with open and arthroscopic treatments but with improved range of motion (ROM) in arthroscopic group.

   d. Risk factors for recurrence:

      i. <20 years of age at the time of surgery

      ii. Participation in contact sports

      iii. Ligamentous laxity

      iv. Glenoid bone loss

      v. Hill-Sachs lesion.

   e. Contraindicated in >25% glenoid bone loss (▶**Fig. 14.3**).

2. HAGL repair:

   a. Missed HAGL lesion may lead to failure of Bankart repair

   b. Can be repaired with open or arthroscopic technique

   c. Suture anchors typically used to repair inferior glenohumeral ligament (IGHL) to its humeral attachment.

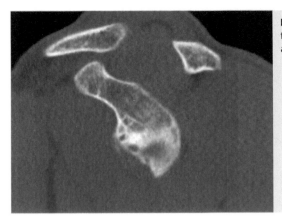

Fig. 14.3 Sagittal computed tomography (CT) showing large anteroinferior bone loss.

F. Procedures for glenoid bone loss:
    1. Bristow-Latarjet procedure:
        a. Transfer of coracoid process to anteroinferior glenoid:
            i.   Traditional fixation with lag screws (▶**Fig. 14.4**)
            ii. Recent literature reports use of suture buttons in some arthroscopic cases.
        b. Used in cases of bone loss or revision but can also be used as primary treatment in cases of anteroinferior instability without bone loss
        c. Achieves stability in three ways:
            i.   Increase glenoid size and translation distance required for dislocation
            ii. Capsule is repaired to the coracoacromial (CA) ligament
            iii. Conjoint tendon provides dynamic sling effect.
        d. Better long-term outcomes than Bankart repair:
            i.   Fewer recurrence
            ii. Higher patient satisfaction.
        e. Higher early complication rate:
            i.   Recurrence or arthrosis due to malpositioning
            ii. Graft fracture or osteolysis
            iii. Neurovascular injury
            iv. Nonunion.
        f. Primarily performed as an open procedure but more recently performed arthroscopically in a few centers.

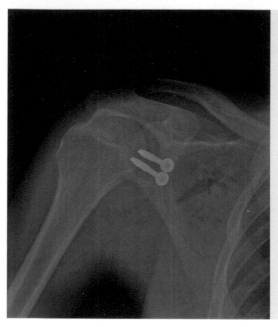

Fig. 14.4 Postoperative radiograph after Latarjet procedure.

2. Eden-Hybinette procedure:
   a. Iliac crest bone block placed anteroinferiorly on glenoid (▶ Fig. 14.5):
      i. Alternatives include iliac crest or distal tibia allograft.
   b. Used in cases of glenoid bone loss or failed Latarjet
   c. Open procedure with some reports of being performed arthroscopically
   d. Higher rates of arthrosis and recurrence than Latarjet with added donor site morbidity.

G. Procedures for humeral (Hill-Sachs) lesions:
   1. Remplissage:
      a. Posterior capsule and rotator cuff fixed into defect to prevent engaging on glenoid
      b. Commonly done concurrently with Bankart repair
      c. Performed arthroscopically and by open procedure but may be easier with arthroscopic approach
      d. May lead to loss of motion.
   2. Humeral head allograft or bone grafting:
      a. For lesions involving >40% of the humeral head
      b. High complication and reoperation rate:
         i. Graft necrosis or resorption
         ii. Arthrosis.
      c. Traditionally an open procedure but has been performed arthroscopically recently.

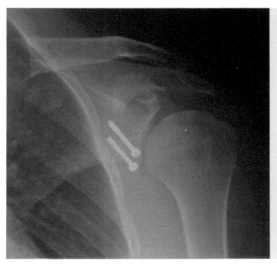

Fig. 14.5 Postoperative radiograph after Eden-Hybinette procedure.

3. Rotational (Weber) osteotomy:
   a. Rotates Hill-Sachs lesion to prevent engagement
   b. High reoperation rate:
      i. Hardware removal
      ii. Nonunion
      iii. Recurrence
      iv. Excessive rotation.

4. Resurfacing/Arthroplasty:
   a. For large lesions
   b. Removes lesion and replaces with implant to prevent engagement
   c. Has outcomes and complications associated with arthroplasty procedures:
      i. Less desirable in younger patients.

5. Other procedures:
   a. Trillat procedure:
      i. Closing wedge osteotomy on undersurface of coracoid process, which is then fixed to glenoid neck with screw
      ii. Primarily open procedure that has been performed arthroscopically
      iii. Performed in patients with concern for graft fracture if Latarjet is performed or if there is concern for nonhealing of labral repair
      iv. Iatrogenic coracoid impingement may lead to loss of motion and arthrosis.
   b. Putti-Platt procedure:
      i. Subscapularis divided with lateral portion fixed to glenoid and medial portion fixed to humerus in a pants over vest fashion
      ii. Results in loss of motion and variable recurrence rates.

II. Posterior instability

A. Much less common than anterior instability:

    1. 2–5% of glenohumeral dislocations.

B. Indications for surgical treatment:

    1. Recurrent instability or symptomatic subluxation after failed conservative treatment.

C. Contraindications:

    1. Voluntary dislocators

    2. Untreated medical condition leading to dislocation (seizure).

D. Associated lesions:

    1. Posterior Bankart:

        a. Soft tissue

        b. Bony.

    2. Reverse Hill-Sachs (▶ **Fig. 14.6**)

    3. Increased glenoid retroversion.

E. Procedures for soft tissue lesions:

    1. Posterior Bankart repair and/or capsular shift:

        a. Similar outcomes for open and arthroscopic procedures

        b. High success rates and good return to sport for isolated posterior instability/laxity.

F. Glenoid bony procedures:

    1. Posterior bone block:

        a. Various graft options:

            i. Iliac crest autograft

            ii. Iliac crest allograft

            iii. Distal tibia allograft

            iv. Scapular spine autograft.

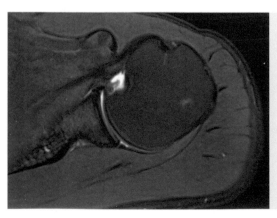

Fig. 14.6 Axial T2 magnetic resonance imaging (MRI) showing reverse Hill-Sachs lesion.

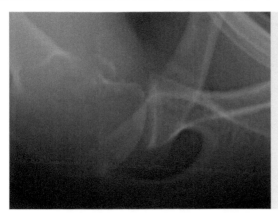

Fig. 14.7 Postoperative axillary radiograph after modified McLaughlin procedure.

    b. Useful in cases of bone loss or revision of soft tissue procedure:

        i. Indications not as clearly defined as in cases of anterior bone loss.

2. Posterior glenoid neck osteotomy:

    a. Opening wedge osteotomy of posterior glenoid neck:

        i. Decreases retroversion of glenoid

        ii. High complication rate

        iii. High rate of arthrosis.

3. Procedures for humeral lesions (Reverse Hill-Sachs):

    a. McLaughlin/Modified McLaughlin

        i. Initially described as transfer of subscapularis into lesion

        ii. Modified procedure uses lesser tuberosity osteotomy (▶ **Fig. 14.7**).

    b. Humeral head allograft or bone grafting:

        i. High complication and reoperation rates

        ii. Traditionally an open procedure but has been performed arthroscopically.

    c. Resurfacing/Arthroplasty

        i. Removes lesion and replaces with implant to prevent engagement

        ii. Outcomes and complications associated with arthroplasty procedures:

           • Less desirable in younger patients.

Suggested Readings

Boileau P, Villalba M, Héry JY, Balg F, Ahrens P, Neyton L. Risk factors for recurrence of shoulder instability after arthroscopic Bankart repair. J Bone Joint Surg Am 2006;88(8):1755–1763

Burkhart SS, De Beer JF. Traumatic glenohumeral bone defects and their relationship to failure of arthroscopic Bankart repairs: significance of the inverted-pear glenoid and the humeral engaging Hill-Sachs lesion. Arthroscopy 2000;16(7):677–694

Fabbriciani C, Milano G, Demontis A, Fadda S, Ziranu F, Mulas PD. Arthroscopic versus open treatment of Bankart lesion of the shoulder: a prospective randomized study. Arthroscopy 2004;20(5):456–462

Fabre T, Abi-Chahla ML, Billaud A, Geneste M, Durandeau A. Long-term results with Bankart procedure: a 26-year follow-up study of 50 cases. J Shoulder Elbow Surg 2010;19(2):318–323

Petrera M, Patella V, Patella S, Theodoropoulos J. A meta-analysis of open versus arthroscopic Bankart repair using suture anchors. Knee Surg Sports Traumatol Arthrosc 2010;18(12):1742–1747

Streubel PN, Krych AJ, Simone JP, et al. Anterior glenohumeral instability: a pathology-based surgical treatment strategy. J Am Acad Orthop Surg 2014;22(5):283–294

Tannenbaum E, Sekiya JK. Evaluation and management of posterior shoulder instability. Sports Health 2011;3(3):253–263

Zimmermann SM, Scheyerer MJ, Farshad M, Catanzaro S, Rahm S, Gerber C. Long-term restoration of anterior shoulder stability: a retrospective analysis of arthroscopic Bankart repair versus open Latarjet procedure. J Bone Joint Surg Am 2016;98(23):1954–1961

15 Osteoarthritis

Matthew Binkley and Joseph Ferraro

Summary

With an ever-aging population, osteoarthritis of the shoulder has become an increasingly prevalent condition for the primary care physician and the orthopaedic surgeon alike. Understanding the pathophysiology and treatment of this condition is a necessary skill for a treating physician. Throughout this chapter, the presentation, diagnosis, and treatment of shoulder osteoarthritis will be presented to aid in appropriate diagnosis and management.

Keywords: Osteoarthritis, glenohumeral arthritis, acromioclavicular arthritis, OA

I. General overview

A. Both glenohumeral and acromioclavicular arthritis are common causes of pain in the shoulder

B. The glenohumeral joint is the third most common joint requiring replacement for end stage arthritis after the hip and knee respectively[1]

C. Primary osteoarthritis is a diagnosis of exclusion as inflammatory arthritis, crystal arthropathy, post-traumatic arthropathy, neuropathic arthropathy, or avascular necrosis can all lead to end stage shoulder arthritis

D. The true incidence of arthritis of the shoulder is unknown:

   1. Glenohumeral arthritis:

      a. More common in women than men

      b. Higher incidence after the age of 60[2]

      c. Increased risk of developing osteoarthritis with past history of shoulder dislocation[3]

      d. Genetic contribution is poorly understood, although primary osteoarthritis of the shoulder is likely due to an interplay between genetic predisposition and environmental factors.[4]

   2. Acromioclavicular arthritis:

      a. More common than glenohumeral arthritis

      b. Common in overhead manual laborers, weight lifters, and overhead athletes

      c. Increased incidence in individuals performing manual labor[5]

      d. Can also be due to a post-traumatic etiology after dislocation or distal clavicle fracture.

E. Clinical symptoms include progressive upper extremity pain, trouble sleeping, and difficulty performing work-related tasks or activities of daily living:

   1. Often complain of deep aching within or on top of the shoulder, and catching or popping with certain motions.

F. Commonly associated conditions include biceps tendonopathy, glenoid bone wear, rotator cuff tear, and labral degeneration:

    1. Rotator cuff tears are often seen in conjunction with arthritis but can be difficult to appreciate clinically due to overall loss of motion and pain with examination maneuvers.

G. Treatment:

    1. Operative and nonoperative management options depending on the degree of disability and loss of function.

II. Anatomy

A. Osteology:

    1. The shoulder consists of the glenohumeral, acromioclavicular, scapulothoracic, and sternoclavicular joints

    2. The shoulder itself is a ball and socket joint consisting of the glenoid medially and the humeral head laterally:

        a. Hyaline cartilage covers the articulating portions of the joint

        b. The humerus is 20–30 degrees retroverted

        c. The glenoid is generally neutral to several degrees retroverted.

    3. The shoulder includes the scapula (the superior portion), the acromion (the articulating portion), the glenoid, and the coracoid process anteriorly:

        a. The coracoid serves as the attachment site for the coracobrachialis, pectoralis minor, coracoclavicular ligaments, coracoacromial ligament, coracohumeral ligament, and the short head of the biceps.

    4. The acromioclavicular joint is a diarthrodial joint

    5. The distal clavicle attaches to the acromion with fibrocartilage joint surfaces and a disc separating the two bony ends with a capsule surrounding the joint.

B. Vasculature:

    1. Blood supply to the humeral head is provided by the posterior and anterior humeral circumflex vessels. The posterior circumflex is believed to provide most of the blood supply:[6]

        a. The ascending branch of the anterior circumflex artery is the arcuate artery, which runs lateral and parallel to the bicipital groove.

        b. Branches of the suprascapular artery also contributes blood supply to the shoulder.

    2. The acromioclavicular joint blood supply derives from the suprascapular artery and the thoracoacromial artery.

C. Nerves:

    1. Shoulder joint:

        a. Axillary nerve

        b. Suprascapular nerve

        c. Lateral pectoral nerve.

2. Acromioclavicular joint:
   a. Suprascapular nerve
   b. Lateral pectoral nerve.

III. Glenohumeral arthritis

A. Definition:
   1. Loss of articular cartilage between the humeral head and glenoid fossa
   2. Diagnosis is made by history and clinical examination in conjunction with radiographs.
B. Clinical presentation:
   1. Age of onset typically in patients older than 50 but can present earlier in patients with a prior traumatic shoulder injury
   2. Common complaints include deep aching in the shoulder that is worse with activity:
      a. May have minimal to no pain at rest.
   3. Difficulty sleeping, especially on the affected shoulder
   4. Normally pain begins with no inciting event and tends to worsen with time
   5. Loss of range of motion (particularly external rotation).
C. Evaluation:
   1. Physical examination:
      a. Neurovascular upper extremity examination:
         i. Sensation, strength, and pulses to rule out cervical spine pathology.
      b. Shoulder examination:
         i. Loss of range of motion passively and actively with end range-of-motion pain
         ii. Forward flexion
         iii. Abduction
         iv. External rotation
         v. Internal rotation (behind the back).
      c. Pain to palpation throughout the shoulder is common. Palpate:
         i. Acromioclavicular joint
         ii. Biceps groove
         iii. Lesser and greater tuberosities
         iv. Acromion
         v. Scapular spine
         vi. Scapular medial border.
      d. Joint effusion is sometimes present
      e. Crepitus with range of motion

f. Anterior shoulder may appear flattened because of posterior subluxation:

    i. It is often difficult to determine the integrity of the rotator cuff secondary to patient's pain with range of motion and overall limitation of range of motion (especially internal and external rotations):

        • Test strength in internal/external rotation, Jobe test.

2. Imaging:

  a. Shoulder radiographs are normally diagnostic:

    i. A full series of shoulder radiographs include an anteroposterior (AP) view, a Grashey view, a lateral (Scapular Y) view, and an axillary view:

        • AP view may show loss of joint space (although this is better visualized in a Grashey view) with osteophytes of the proximal humerus or loose bodies. The humeral head should be concentric within the glenoid (▶ **Fig. 15.1**).

        • Grashey view is the true AP view of the shoulder and best shows the glenohumeral joint.

        • Axillary view should be examined to determine wear of the glenoid. Often the humeral head is posteriorly subluxed in osteoarthritis.

        • Scapular Y view is helpful to identify locations of loose bodies and to evaluate the bony architecture of the shoulder further.

    ii. Features common to osteoarthritis of the shoulder include loss of joint space, loose bodies, osteophytes along the humeral head (goat's beard), subchondral cysts, and glenoid bone loss which is generally posterior and often accompanied by posterior humeral head subluxation.

  b. Further evaluation of the glenohumeral joint bone structure can be done with a computed tomography (CT) imaging series to examine the degree of arthritis present and rotator cuff integrity versus a magnetic resonance imaging (MRI) which better visualizes the rotator cuff at the expense of bone detail.

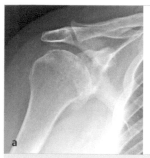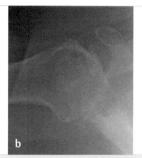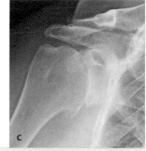

Fig. 15.1 (a–c) Ateroposterior (AP), axillary, and Grashey views of an arthritic shoulder showing osteophyte formation along the inferior humeral head, cysts within the humeral head, and lack of joint space with retroversion of the glenoid.

3. Classification:

    a. Walch classification system of glenoid bone wear is commonly used (►**Table 15.1**).

D. Treatment:

    1. Nonoperative:

        a. Avoidance of activities that exacerbate pain

        b. Physical therapy and at-home stretching with goal to maintain range of motion and strength of periscapular muscles

        c. Ice or heat

        d. Medications:

            i. Nonsteroidal anti-inflammatory drugs

            ii. Acetaminophen

            iii. Oral steroid dose pack.

        e. Corticosteroid joint injections versus joint lubrication injections (hyaluronic acid) versus biologics (minimal evidence of efficacy).

    2. Operative:

        a. Surgery is indicated when nonoperative measures fail

        b. Treatment depends on patient factors which include age, degree of glenoid bone wear, glenoid version, medical comorbidities, associated pathology (i.e., rotator cuff tears), and work status

Table 15.1 Modified Walsh classification

Type A Concentric wear with a well-centered humeral head	A1 Minor central erosion of the glenoid
	A2 Deep central erosion with line connecting the anterior and posterior glenoid bisecting the humeral head
Type B Asymmetric posterior glenoid wear with posterior subluxation of the humeral head	B1 Posterior joint space narrowing with no posterior bone loss
	B2 Biconcave glenoid with retroversion of the glenoid and bone loss present
	B3 Posterior wear with retroversion >15 degrees or humeral head subluxation >70%
Type C Dysplastic glenoid retroversion present	Glenoid retroversion of >25 degrees
Type D	Glenoid anteversion or anterior humeral head subluxation

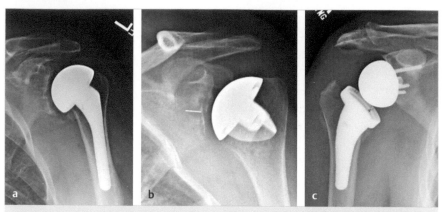

Fig. 15.2 (a, b) Types of total shoulder arthroplasty with a polyethylene glenoid component cemented into place. (c) Reverse shoulder arthroplasty where the ball and socket are reversed to help improve joint kinematics and motion with rotator cuff pathology is present.

    c. In early arthritis, arthroscopic debridement and capsular releases can be performed:

        i. Modest early results are common, with a high reoperation rate in both the short and long terms.[7]

    d. Hemiarthroplasty is considered in young patients with end stage arthritis or patients with severe glenoid bone loss with an intact rotator cuff:

        i. Hemiarthroplasty has a higher revision rate than primary total shoulder arthroplasty secondary to pain from glenoid-sided arthrosis, which commonly develops.[8]

    e. The most effective treatment for advanced arthritis of the glenohumeral joint is total shoulder arthroplasty, in which the glenoid and humeral head are resurfaced with metal and polyethylene. Anatomic total shoulder arthroplasty is the traditional treatment for shoulder arthritis but there are increasing indications for which reverse shoulder arthroplasty is more appropriate due to severe bone wear or accompanying pathology. Total shoulder arthroplasty requires the rotator cuff to be intact (▶ Fig. 15.2):

        i. Among patients who undergo total shoulder arthroplasty, 90% experience complete or nearly complete pain relief with improved range of motion after surgery.[8]

IV. Acromioclavicular joint (ACJ) arthritis

A. Definition:

    1. Loss of joint space with osteophytes and subchondral cysts common

    2. Diagnosis is made based on clinical examination in conjunction with radiographic evidence of osteoarthritis.

B. Clinical presentation:

    1. Occurs most commonly in the 3rd and 4th decades of life

    2. Common in overhead workers, weight lifters, and manual laborers

3. Pain may be focal to the ACJ without radiation, or it may produce symptoms of vague neck and shoulder pain

4. Pain with overhead or cross-body activities

5. Pain at night while sleeping on affected shoulder.

C. Evaluation:

    1. Physical examination:

        a. Patients often point to their ACJ as the source of their pain

        b. Active and passive motion of the shoulder often remain intact

        c. Examine the shoulder bilaterally to evaluate for deformity at the ACJ

        d. ACJ is typically tender to palpation. Compare with the contralateral side to ensure any tenderness to palpation is related to the symptoms the patient is experiencing as deep palpation of the ACJ may be uncomfortable even in asymptomatic patients

        e. Cross-body adduction test: Shoulder is flexed to 90 degrees and adducted across the body, with pain reproduced in the ACJ considered positive

        f. Active compression test (O'Brien's test): The arm is flexed forward to 90 degrees and adducted 10 degrees with resisted pronation. This maneuver is repeated with resisted supination of the forearm. Pain with pronation that is relieved by supination is a positive test for ACJ pathology.

    2. Imaging:

        a. Standard shoulder radiographs are normally adequate to view the ACJ (▶ **Fig. 15.3**):

            i. Zanca view is a 15 degrees cephalad view that provides the best view of the ACJ (▶ **Fig. 15.4**)

            ii. Radiographs can be misleading as not all patients with radiographic signs of arthritis manifest symptoms; some patients with normal radiographs have symptoms related to joint-space wear in the ACJ.[9]

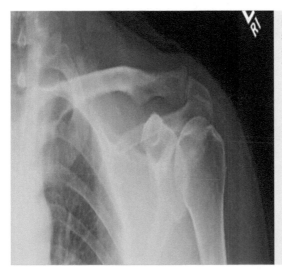

Fig. 15.3 Radiograph of the left shoulder indicating distal clavicle arthritis with cyst formation and osteophytes present.

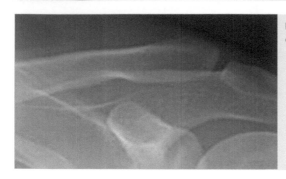

Fig. 15.4 Zanca view of the left clavicle.

    b. MRI is not needed routinely for isolated ACJ arthritis but can be helpful when confounding factors are present. On MRI, ACJ arthrosis may show edema in the distal clavicle and proximal acromion in symptomatic patients, which can aid in the diagnosis. ACJ arthritis is also common with other shoulder disorders, which may require MRI for definitive diagnosis (▶ **Fig. 15.5**)

    c. Ultrasonography can show osteophytes and joint-space narrowing and can be helpful for joint arthrocentesis. Ultrasound as a diagnostic tool is rarely used however.

D. Treatment:

    1. Nonoperative:

        a. Nonsteroidal anti-inflammatory medications

        b. Acetaminophen

        c. ACJ corticosteroid injection:

            i. Intra-articular ACJ injections have variable results but often provide short-term relief and improvement in range of motion[10]

            ii. Helpful as a diagnostic tool if the diagnosis is doubtful.

    2. Operative:

        a. Distal clavicle excision:

            i. Performed arthroscopically or in an open surgical fashion

            ii. Good outcomes have been reported after open or arthroscopic surgery[11]

            iii. Results have been less predictable in cases involving worker's compensation or litigation, or heavy manual laborers

            iv. The most common complication is continued pain, which is often caused by inadequate resection

            v. ACJ instability can occur postoperatively if resection of the distal clavicle is too aggressive.

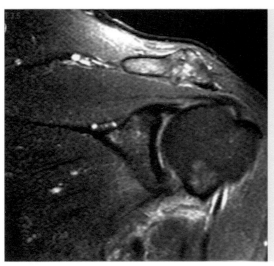

Fig. 15.5 Magnetic resonance imaging (MRI) of the left clavicle showing edema in the distal clavicle and proximal acromion indicative of distal clavicle arthritis.

Suggested Readings

Alluri RK, Kupperman AI, Montgomery SR, Wang JC, Hame SL. Demographic analysis of open and arthroscopic distal clavicle excision in a private insurance database. Arthroscopy 2014;30(9):1068–1074

Oh JH, Kim JY, Choi JH, Park SM. Is arthroscopic distal clavicle resection necessary for patients with radiological acromioclavicular joint arthritis and rotator cuff tears? A prospective randomized comparative study. Am J Sports Med 2014;42(11):2567–2573

Park YB, Koh KH, Shon MS, Park YE, Yoo JC. Arthroscopic distal clavicle resection in symptomatic acromioclavicular joint arthritis combined with rotator cuff tear: a prospective randomized trial. Am J Sports Med 2015;43(4):985–990

Roberson TA, Bentley JC, Griscom JT, et al. Outcomes of total shoulder arthroplasty in patients younger than 65 years: a systematic review. J Shoulder Elbow Surg 2017;26(7):1298–1306

Sayegh ET, Mascarenhas R, Chalmers PN, Cole BJ, Romeo AA, Verma NN. Surgical treatment options for glenohumeral arthritis in young patients: a systematic review and meta-analysis. Arthroscopy 2015;31(6):1156–1166.e8

Sowa B, Bochenek M, Bülhoff M, et al. The medium- and long-term outcome of total shoulder arthroplasty for primary glenohumeral osteoarthritis in middle-aged patients. Bone Joint J 2017;99-B(7):939–943

Trofa D, Rajaee SS, Smith EL. Nationwide trends in total shoulder arthroplasty and hemiarthroplasty for osteoarthritis. Am J Orthop 2014;43(4):166–172

References

1. Australian Orthopaedic Association National Joint Replacement Registry. 2016 Annual report. https://aoanjrr.sahmri.com/documents/10180/275066/Hip%2C%20Knee%20%26%20Shoulder%20Arthroplasty. Accessed on November 17, 2017

2. Kobayashi T, Takagishi K, Shitara H, et al. Prevalence of and risk factors for shoulder osteoarthritis in Japanese middle-aged and elderly populations. J Shoulder Elbow Surg 2014;23(5):613–619

3. Plath JE, Aboalata M, Seppel G, et al. Prevalence of and risk factors for dislocation arthropathy: radiological long-term outcome of arthroscopic Bankart repair in 100 shoulders at an average 13-year follow-up. Am J Sports Med 2015;43(5):1084–1090

4. Casagrande D, Stains JP, Murthi AM. Identification of shoulder osteoarthritis biomarkers: comparison between shoulders with and without osteoarthritis. J Shoulder Elbow Surg 2015;24(3):382–390

5. Svendsen SW, Gelineck J, Egund N, Frost P. 0215 Acromioclavicular joint degeneration in relation to cumulative occupational mechanical exposures: a magnetic resonance imaging study. Occup Environ Med 2014;71(1):A28

6. Hettrich CM, Boraiah S, Dyke JP, Neviaser A, Helfet DL, Lorich DG. Quantitative assessment of the vascularity of the proximal part of the humerus. J Bone Joint Surg Am 2010;92(4):943–948

7. Sayegh ET, Mascarenhas R, Chalmers PN, Cole BJ, Romeo AA, Verma NN. Surgical treatment options for glenohumeral arthritis in young patients: a systematic review and meta-analysis. Arthroscopy 2015;31(6):1156–1166.e8

8. Eichinger JK, Miller LR, Hartshorn T, Li X, Warner JJ, Higgins LD. Evaluation of satisfaction and durability after hemiarthroplasty and total shoulder arthroplasty in a cohort of patients aged 50 years or younger: an analysis of discordance of patient satisfaction and implant survival. J Shoulder Elbow Surg 2016;25(5):772–780

9. Elhassan B, Ozbaydar M, Diller D, Massimini D, Higgins LD, Warner JJ. Open versus arthroscopic acromioclavicular joint resection: a retrospective comparison study. Arthroscopy 2009;25(11):1224–1232

10. Park KD, Kim TK, Lee J, Lee WY, Ahn JK, Park Y. Palpation versus ultrasound-guided acromioclavicular joint intra-articular corticosteroid injections: a retrospective comparative clinical study. Pain Physician 2015;18(4):333–341

11. Mall NA, Foley E, Chalmers PN, Cole BJ, Romeo AA, Bach BR Jr. Degenerative joint disease of the acromioclavicular joint: a review. Am J Sports Med 2013;41(11):2684–2692

16 Total Shoulder Arthroplasty

Matthew Baker and Uma Srikumaran

Summary

Shoulder replacement has its origins in France in 1893. Since then, there have been many advances in the implant and technique for shoulder arthroplasty. It has been estimated that the demand for total shoulder replacement will increase by 755% between 2011 and 2030.[1]

Keywords: Total shoulder arthroplasy, shoulder replacement, shoulder arthritis, TSA

I. Indications

A. Osteoarthritis

B. Rheumatoid arthritis

C. Avascular necrosis

D. Posttraumatic arthritis

E. Postinstability arthropathy

F. Pain that has failed to respond to conservative measures

G. Functional decline that is unacceptable to the patient

H. Postinfectious arthropathy.[2]

II. Contraindications

A. Absolute:

   1. Active infection.

B. Relative:

   1. Rotator cuff (RTC)/deltoid dysfunction

      a. Irreparable tear, paralysis, and other previous injury

      b. Previous surgery involving take down/repair of the subscapularis.

   2. Neuropathic joint:

      a. Charcot and syringomyelia.

   3. Severe brachial plexopathy

   4. Approach those with prior infection cautiously

   5. Intractable instability.

III. Presentation/Evaluation

A. Insidious onset of pain, which is slowly progressive

B. Progressive stiffness

C. Functional limitations:
   1. Activities of daily living (ADLs)
   2. Hobbies.
D. Medical problems
E. For those with avascular necrosis (AVN):
   1. Attempt to determine the cause
   2. Evaluate other joints.

IV. Physical examination (PE)

A. Range of motion (ROM):
   1. Active and passive
   2. Osteoarthritis (OA) and AVN:
      a. Global motion loss, particularly external rotation (ER).
B. RTC strength:
   1. Can be difficult to ascertain due to pain.
C. Cervical examination
D. Neurovascular examination
E. Pain localization
F. Evaluate for instability
G. Scapulothoracic motion and lag signs

V. Imaging

Plain radiographs are most important:
A. Anteroposterior (AP):
   1. Inferior osteophytes
   2. Humeral canal diameter
   3. Acromiohumeral distance:
      a. Less than 6 mm strongly suggestive of RTC tear.
B. Axillary:
   1. Glenoid version
   2. Glenoid wear
   3. Posterior subluxation.
C. Definitive assessment of glenoid version and bone stock:
   1. Can glenoid be resurfaced?
      a. Medialization of the glenoid past the coracoid → Don't resurface the glenoid.
   2. Treat 15-degree posterior glenoid wear with anterior glenoid reaming 50% change of a successful correction[3]
   3. Bone graft needed?
   4. Walch classification.[4]

D. Magnetic resonance imaging (MRI):
1. Can be used if RTC tear is suspected:
   a. Uncommon with OA
   b. RTC tear of 5 to 10% at the time of total shoulder arthroplasty.
2. May be used if acromiohumeral distance decreased or in case of prior cuff surgery
3. Also used to stage AVN.

VI. Approach

A. Deltopectoral:
1. Uses the deltopectoral interval
2. Provides excellent exposure for the proximal humerus
3. Detach subscapularis and anterior capsule:
   a. Lesser tuberosity osteotomy (LTO) versus peel versus tenotomy
   b. No current evidence that one approach is significantly better than another.
4. Need to do capsular releases for glenoid exposure
5. Risks:
   a. Axillary nerve
   b. Cephalic vein.

B. Superior:
1. Splits the deltoid
2. Excellent humeral exposure
3. Using this approach may decrease instability as the subscapularis is not violated[5]
4. Risks:
   a. Glenoid component malpositioning
   b. Axillary nerve injury.

C. Technical considerations:
1. Glenoid component: Pegged versus keeled, cemented, metal backed:
   a. Avoid use of metal-backed glenoid components as they have high failure rate
   b. Lower incidence of radiolucent lines in pegged design
   c. It is not known if there is any clinical difference in the implant designs.
2. Humeral stem can be cemented, cementless, or stemless:
   a. Position in 25 to 45 degrees retroversion
   b. Top of the humeral head shoulder be 5 to 8 mm above the greater tuberosity.
3. Want to recreate anatomy:
   a. Challenges include glenoid wear, especially posterior, increased glenoid retroversion, and limited bone stock.
4. Avoid over resection of the humeral head.

    D.   Avoid iatrogenic RTC injury during humeral head osteotomy

    E.   Postoperative rehabilitation should focus on minimizing tension on the subscapularis repair:

        1.   Focus on passive range of motion and active assist range of motion, limiting passive external rotation.

VII. Results

    A.   Pain relief:

        1.   Most predictable benefit

        2.   More than 90% can be expected to attain good pain relief

        3.   Most who don't have an explainable cause:

            a.   Intraoperative complication

            b.   Postoperative complication.

        4.   Better results when compared to hemiarthroplasty with improved pain relief, functional outcomes, and patient satisfaction.[6]

    B.   Survival:

        1.   93 to 97% at 10 years

        2.   84% at 20 years

        3.   Can be dependent on indication for surgery:

            a.   61% at 10 years when done after previous instability procedure.[7]

VIII. Complications

    A.   Loosening:

        1.   Glenoid:

            a.   Most common reason for reoperation.

        2.   Humeral component loosening is suggestive of prosthetic joint infection:

            a.   Uncommon

            b.   Think infection.

    B.   Instability:

        1.   Subscapularis failure

        2.   Glenoid loosening.

    C.   Fracture:

        1.   Intraoperative: 1.5%

        2.   Treat tuberosity fractures with reduction and suture fixation

        3.   Treat shaft fractures with long stem and cerclage wires

        4.   Postoperative:

            a.   Wright and Cofield classification of periprosthetic fracture.

D. Infection:
   1. Rate: 2 to 3%
   2. Workup includes complete blood count, erythrocyte sedimentation rate, C-reactive protein, joint aspiration, and arthroscopic tissue sampling
   3. Must hold cultures for at least 15 days to eval for Cutibacterium acnes
   4. Irrigation/debridement versus two-stage revision.

IX. Revision

A. Timing of symptoms (early vs. late):
   1. Early:
      a. Pain—infection and malpositioned components
      b. Stiffness—component malposition and capsular contracture
      c. Loss of strength—nerve injury
      d. Instability—mispositioned components, nerve injury, and subscapularis repair failure.
   2. Late:
      a. Pain—infection and component loosening
      b. Stiffness—poor compliance with rehabilitation and pain
      c. Loss of strength—RTC tears, poor rehabilitation, and loss of tuberosities
      d. Instability—cuff deficiency and glenoid wear.
B. Must know indication for index procedure, details of previous surgeries, and rehabilitation protocol
C. Pay careful attention to:
   1. Passive and active ROM
   2. RTC strength
   3. Muscle atrophy
   4. Subscapularis function
   5. Look for superior escape.
D. Also consider other possible pain etiologies:
   1. AC pathology, biceps pathology, cervical spine, scapulothoracic, and thoracic outlet.

X. Reasons for failure

A. Soft tissue deficiencies:
   1. Deltoid scarring/detachment
   2. Anterior capsule scarring and subscapularis scarring
   3. Cuff insufficiency.

B. Bone deficiencies:

1. Glenoid or proximal humerus

2. Often lead to instability.

C. Component loosening:

1. Glenoid much more common:

   a. Can be related to malpositioning of the components.

2. Abnormal joint mechanics, increased component stress causing cement mantle fracture resulting in glenoid loosening and ultimate failure.

XI. Imaging workup

A. X-ray—standard shoulder series:

1. Assess for component positioning, bone loss, loosening, or migration

2. Evaluate sequential radiographs.

B. Computed tomography (CT) scan:

1. Assess component version and bone loss.

C. Bone scan:

1. Can be used to evaluate for loosening.

D. Expected outcomes of revision can be based on indication:

1. Component revisions do better than soft tissue reconstructions

2. Best outcomes:

   a. Periprosthetic open reduction internal fixation

   b. Implantation or revision of glenoid component.

3. Tuberosity reconstruction, hemiarthroplasty for cuff tear arthropathy, and infections have bad outcomes.

Suggested Readings

Bhat SB, Lazarus M, Getz C, Williams GR Jr, Namdari S. Economic decision model suggests total shoulder arthroplasty is superior to hemiarthroplasty in young patients with end-stage shoulder arthritis. Clin Orthop Relat Res 2016;474(11):2482–2492

Brolin TJ, Thakar OV, Abboud JA. Outcomes after shoulder replacement surgery in the young patient: how do they do and how long can we expect them to last? Clin Sports Med 2018;37(4):593–607

Hernandez NM, Chalmers BP, Wagner ER, Sperling JW, Cofield RH, Sanchez-Sotelo J. Revision to reverse total shoulder arthroplasty restores stability for patients with unstable shoulder prostheses. Clin Orthop Relat Res 2017;475(11):2716–2722

Johnson DJ, Johnson CC, Gulotta LV. Return to play after shoulder replacement surgery: what is realistic and what does the evidence tell us. Clin Sports Med 2018;37(4):585–592

Lazarus MD, Cox RM, Murthi AM, Levy O, Abboud JA. Stemless prosthesis for total shoulder arthroplasty. J Am Acad Orthop Surg 2017;25(12):e291–e300

Padegimas EM, Nicholson TA, Silva S, et al. Outcomes of shoulder arthroplasty performed for postinfectious arthritis. Clin Orthop Surg 2018;10(3):344–351

Roberson TA, Bentley JC, Griscom JT, et al. Outcomes of total shoulder arthroplasty in patients younger than 65 years: a systematic review. J Shoulder Elbow Surg 2017;26(7):1298–1306

Service BC, Hsu JE, Somerson JS, Russ SM, Matsen FA III. Does postoperative glenoid retroversion affect the 2-year clinical and radiographic outcomes for total shoulder arthroplasty? Clin Orthop Relat Res 2017;475(11):2726–2739

Simovitch R, Flurin PH, Marczuk Y, et al. Rate of improvement in clinical outcomes with anatomic and reverse total shoulder arthroplasty. Bull Hosp Jt Dis (2013) 2015;73(Suppl 1):S111–S117

Sperling JW, Antuna SA, Sanchez-Sotelo J, Schleck C, Cofield RH. Shoulder arthroplasty for arthritis after instability surgery. J Bone Joint Surg Am 2002;84(10):1775–1781

Torchia ME, Cofield RH, Settergren CR. Total shoulder arthroplasty with the Neer prosthesis: long-term results. J Shoulder Elbow Surg 1997;6(6):495–505

References

1. Padegimas EM, Maltenfort M, Lazarus MD, Ramsey ML, Williams GR, Namdari S. Future patient demand for shoulder arthroplasty by younger patients: national projections. Clin Orthop Relat Res 2015;473(6):1860–1867

2. Padegimas EM, Nicholson TA, Silva S, et al. Outcomes of shoulder arthroplasty performed for postinfectious arthritis. Clin Orthop Surg 2018;10(3):344–351

3. Gillespie R, Lyons R, Lazarus M. Eccentric reaming in total shoulder arthroplasty: a cadaveric study. Orthopedics. 2009;32(1)

4. Bercik MJ, Kruse K, Yalizis M, Gauci M-O, Chaoui J, Walch G. A modification to the Walch classification of the glenoid in primary glenohumeral osteoarthritis using three-dimensional imaging. J Shoulder Elbow Surg 2016;25(10):1601–1606

5. Molé D, Wein F, Dézaly C, Valenti P, Sirveaux F. Surgical technique: the anterosuperior approach for reverse shoulder arthroplasty. Clin Orthop Relat Res 2011;469(9):2461–2468

6. Radnay CS, Setter KJ, Chambers L, Levine WN, Bigliani LU, Ahmad CS. Total shoulder replacement compared with humeral head replacement for the treatment of primary glenohumeral osteoarthritis: a systematic review. J Shoulder Elbow Surg 2007;16(4):396–402

7. Sperling JW, Antuna SA, Sanchez-Sotelo J, Schleck C, Cofield RH. Shoulder arthroplasty for arthritis after instability surgery. J Bone Joint Surg Am 2002;84(10):1775–1781

17 Reverse Total Shoulder Arthroplasty

Matthew Baker and Uma Srikumaran

Summary

The reverse shoulder prosthesis was developed to address issues encountered while treating end stage glenohumeral arthritis in the setting of rotator cuff deficiency. Indications have since expanded to address multiple pathologies of the shoulder.

Keywords: Reverse shoulder arthroplasty, cuff tear arthropathy, arthritis, biomechanics

I. Indications[1]

A. Cuff tear arthropathy (Hamada classification; ▶Fig. 17.1):

1. Degenerative changes associated with massive rotator cuff tears

2. Attempting anatomic replacement in the setting of massive rotator cuff tears leads to failure.

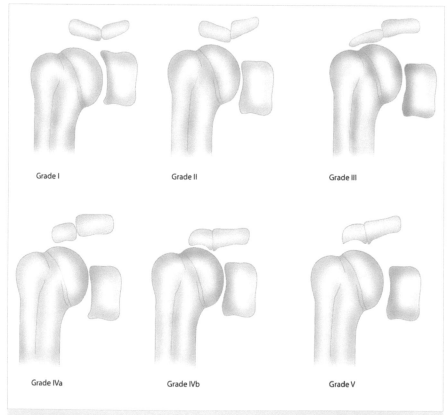

Grade I   Grade II   Grade III

Grade IVa   Grade IVb   Grade V

Fig. 17.1 Hamada classification. Grade I, normal acromialhumeral interval (AHI); Grade II, narrowed AHI <5mm; Grade III, acetabularization of the acromion and narrowing of the AHI; Grade IVa, narrowing of AHI with glenohumeral (GH) narrowing; Grade IVb, AHI and GH narrowing with acetabularization of acromion; Grade V, flattening of the humeral head.

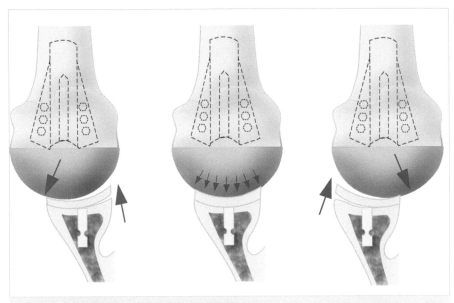

Fig. 17.2 Rocking horse phenomenon.

B. Rocking horse phenomenon (▶ **Fig. 17.2**):

    1. Loss of centralization of the humeral head results in eccentric wear and early failure.

C. Pseudoparalysis:[2,3]

    1. Massive rotator cuff tear with minimal to no arthritis:

        a. Anterior superior escape

        b. There may be improvement in range of motion (ROM) but may not return to full.

    2. Immunologic arthritis

    3. Failed rotator cuff repair

    4. Proximal humeral fractures

    5. Malunions/Nonunions

    6. Revision of anatomic shoulder arthroplasty/hemiarthroplasty

    7. Instability or chronic dislocations

    8. Tumors.

In the United States and Australia more than 50% of reverse arthroplasties are done for arthritis and fracture. In the UK, the majority are done for cuff tear arthropathy including massive rotator cuff tears.[4]

II. Contraindications[1]

A. Nonfunctioning deltoid

B. Axillary nerve injury/damage

C. Active infection

D. Neuropathic joints

E. Glenoid vault deficiency precluding baseplate fixation.

III. Evaluation

A. History:

1. Traumatic versus atraumatic

2. Degree of pain and dysfunction (perceived weakness, instability)

3. Functional demands and expectations

4. Ambulation status (use of assistive devices)

5. Metal allergies

6. Neck pain, alternative origins of pain.

B. Physical examination:

1. Cervical examination

2. Neurovascular examination

3. Pain localization

4. Passive, active motion

5. Strength, stability

6. Evaluate rotator cuff, scapulothoracic motion, lag signs

7. Painless weakness is likely neurologic in origin[5]

8. Hornblower's sign: Indicates torn teres minor and will likely need tendon transfer to regain full motion.

C. Imaging:

1. X-ray:

a. Grashey and axillary at minimum (▶ **Fig. 17.3**).

2. Computed tomography (CT):

a. Evaluate glenoid version, humeral and glenoid bone stock, alignment, and rotator cuff atrophy.

3. Magnetic resonance imaging (MRI):

a. Evaluate glenoid version, humeral and glenoid bone stock, alignment, and rotator cuff atrophy

b. Typically CT or MRI is used. Both modalities are usually not necessary.

IV. Approach

A. Deltopectoral:

1. Subscapular repair based on implant selection.

B. Superior:

1. Split the deltoid

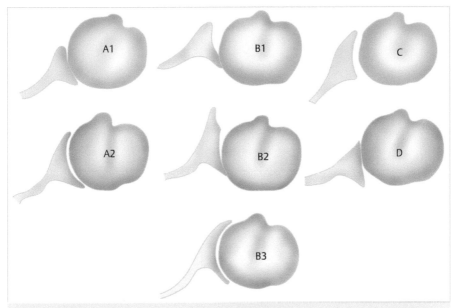

Fig. 17.3 Walch classification. A1, well centered with minor erosion; A2, well centered with major erosion; B1, posterior humeral head subluxation; B2, biconcave glenoid; B3, monocave glenoid preferentially worn posterior with >15 degrees glenoid retroversion or humeral head subluxation of 70%; C, dysplastic >25 degrees retroversion; D, anterior humeral head subluxation or glenoid anteversion.

    2. Technical challenges:
        a. Exposure, glenosphere tilt, axillary nerve injury
        b. Can lead to improved stability as not violating the subscapularis if intact.[6]

V. Types of implants (▶Fig. 17.4 and ▶Fig. 17.5)

A. Grammont:
    1. Medialized center of rotation (COR) (at the glenoid–component interface)
    2. Decreased shear force on the glenoid–component interface
    3. Encroachment on the glenoid → scapular notching
    4. Less mechanical advantage
    5. Laxity of intact rotator cuff.

B. "Lateralized":
    1. Still medial to the anatomic COR, just less so than the Grammont style
    2. More than a hemisphere
    3. Address the issues associated with medialized components
    4. Less scapular notching

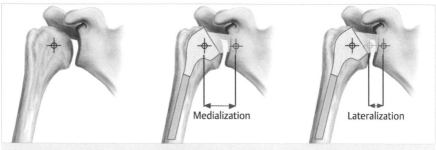

Fig. 17.4 Comparison of the center of rotation.

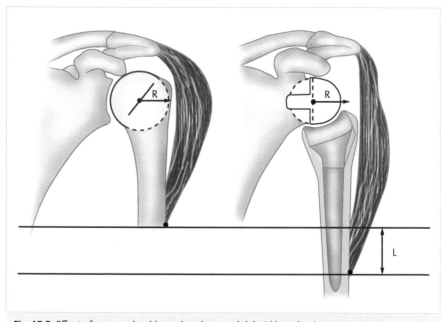

Fig. 17.5 Effect of reverse shoulder arthroplasty and deltoid lengthening.

5. Improved soft tissue tensioning → Increased compressive forces → Decreased instability
6. More force across the glenoid–component interface.

C. Neck shaft angle (NSA) (►**Fig. 17.6**):

1. Normal: 30–55
2. RSA: 125–155
3. More horizontal NSA:
   a. Decreased scapular notching
   b. Increased contact stress → Increased wear
   c. iImproved adduction, external rotation, and extension.[7]

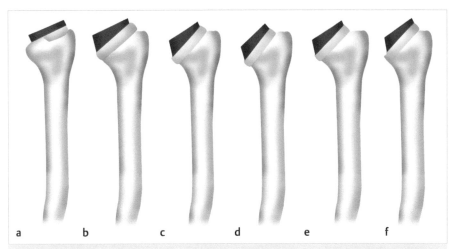

Fig. 17.6 (a–f) Effect of humeral stem design on humeral position and range of motion in reverse shoulder arthroplasty.[7]

D. Glenosphere positioning:[8–10]

    1. Avoid superior tilt

    2. Inferior positioning can decrease scapular notching

    3. Use glenoid center line as reference

    4. Use larger glenosphere for instability.

VI. Outcomes

A. Depends on indication

B. Best results in treating cuff tear arthropathy

C. Use caution in younger patients:

    1. Unknown long-term outcomes in patients less than 70, early results are promising

    2. Use in revision procedures show improvement in pain scores and functional outcomes; results are not as good when compared with use in a primary fracture setting.[11]

D. Implant survivorship:[12,13]

    1. At 10 years 90–93% when looking at revision surgery

    2. At 10 years 90% when looking at Constant score less than 30; decline in Constant score after 9 years (▶ **Table 17.1**).

E. Complications:[1,14,15]

    1. Scapular notching[16] (classification) (▶ **Fig. 17.7**):

        a. Reported rates: 0–96%

        b. Most common and unique complication of RSA

        c. May be implant related → decreased with lateralized components?

        d. There is controversy regarding the clinical relevance of scapular notching.

Table 17.1 Results of RTSA in cuff tear arthropathy

Study	No. of patients	Mean age, year	Mean (range) Follow-up, months	Constant Murely (CM) score		ASES score		Complication rate, %	Reoperation rate, %
				Initial	Final	Initial	Final		
Frankle et al[17]	60	71	33 (24–68)	NR	NR	34	68	22	13
Seebauer et al[18]	57	70	18 (3–44)	NR	67	NR	NR	9	NR
Boileau et al[19]	21	77	40 (24–72)	18	66	NR	76	19	5
Wall et al[20]	59	73	40 (24–86)	22	65	NR	NR	NR	NR
Cuff et al[21]	94	72	28 (24–88)	NR	NR	30	86	9.5	5
Cuff et al[22]	74	70	62 (60–79)	NR	NR	32	75	13.5	NR
Ferreira Neto et al[23]	13	62	53 (32–74)	NR	NR	23	82	15	NR

Abbreviations: ASES, American Shoulder and Elbow Surgeons; CM, Constant-Murley; NR, not reported; RTSA, reverse total shoulder arthroplasty.

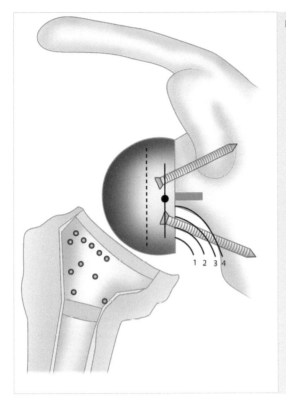

Fig. 17.7 Scapular notching.

F. Instability:[14]
1. Reported rate is 0–31%
2. Component malposition
3. Implant selection → Impingement
4. Soft tissue imbalance
5. Component loosening
6. Infection
7. Early dislocation (<3 months) patient trauma versus inadequate tension
8. Dislocations should be reduced; recurrent instability indication for revision
9. Aseptic base plate loosening:
   a. 3.5–5%
   b. Most common cause is poor initial fixation.

G. Infection:
1. Rate: 1–15%, higher than in anatomic shoulder arthroplasty[1,15]
2. Meta-analysis: 3–5% infection risk
3. Most patients will not have constitution symptoms

4. Many false negative results:

   a. Culture (Cx), erythrocyte sedimentation rate (ESR), C-reactive protein (CRP)

   b. *Cutibacterium acnes* hold for at least 14 days.

5. Acute infection (<6 weeks from surgery): Irrigation and debridement (I&D), poly exchange

6. Chronic infection (>6 weeks from surgery): One- versus two-stage revision:

   a. Prosthesis removal, irrigation and debridement, and antibiotic spacer insertion

   b. Followed by a minimum 6-week course of parenteral, culture specific antibiotics, and re-implantation of the implant.

H. Nerve injury:

   1. Rate: 1.5–24%:

      a. In total shoulder arthroplasty (TSA) 2.2–20%.

   2. Most common is partial brachial plexus lesion

   3. Most common individual nerve is axillary.[15]

I. Intraoperative fracture:

   1. Rate: 1–2%.

J. Component dissociation:

   1. Rate: Reported <1%.

K. Revision procedures have a higher complication rate compared with primary reverse arthroplasty.[15]

References

1. Familiari F, Rojas J, Nedim Doral M, Huri G, McFarland EG. Reverse total shoulder arthroplasty. EFORT Open Rev 2018;3(2):58–69

2. Hyun YS, Huri G, Garbis NG, McFarland EG. Uncommon indications for reverse total shoulder arthroplasty. Clin Orthop Surg 2013;5(4):243–255

3. Mulieri P, Dunning P, Klein S, Pupello D, Frankle M. Reverse shoulder arthroplasty for the treatment of irreparable rotator cuff tear without glenohumeral arthritis. J Bone Joint Surg Am 2010;92(15):2544–2556

4. Singhal K, Rammohan R. Going forward with reverse shoulder arthroplasty. J Clin Orthop Trauma 2018;9(1):87–93

5. McFarland EG. Edward Examination of the Shoulder: The Complete Guide. Thieme Medical Publishers Inc; 2006;1–7

6. Molé D, Wein F, Dézaly C, Valenti P, Sirveaux F. Surgical technique: the anterosuperior approach for reverse shoulder arthroplasty. Clin Orthop Relat Res 2011;469(9):2461–2468

7. Lädermann A, Denard PJ, Boileau P, et al. Effect of humeral stem design on humeral position and range of motion in reverse shoulder arthroplasty. Int Orthop 2015;39(11):2205–2213

8. Keener JD, Patterson BM, Orvets N, Aleem AW, Chamberlain AM. Optimizing reverse shoulder arthroplasty component position in the setting of advanced arthritis with posterior glenoid erosion: a computer-enhanced range of motion analysis. J Shoulder Elbow Surg 2018;27(2):339–349

9. Li X, Knutson Z, Choi D, et al. Effects of glenosphere positioning on impingement-free internal and external rotation after reverse total shoulder arthroplasty. J Shoulder Elbow Surg 2013;22(6):807–813

10. Ackland DC, Patel M, Knox D. Prosthesis design and placement in reverse total shoulder arthroplasty. J Orthop Surg Res 2015;10:101

11. Nikola C, Hrvoje K, Nenad M. Int Orthop 2015;39:343 (SICOT)
12. Bacle G, Nové-Josserand L, Garaud P, Walch G. Long-term outcomes of reverse total shoulder arthroplasty: a follow-up of a previous study. J Bone Joint Surg Am 2017;99(6):454–461
13. Cuff DJ, Pupello DR, Santoni BG, Clark RE, Frankle MA. Reverse shoulder arthroplasty for the treatment of rotator cuff deficiency: a concise follow-up, at a minimum of 10 years, of previous reports. J Bone Joint Surg Am 2017;99(22):1895–1899
14. Bohsali KI, Bois AJ, Wirth MA. Complications of shoulder arthroplasty. J Bone Joint Surg Am 2017;99(3):256–269
15. Barco R, Savvidou OD, Sperling JW, Sanchez-Sotelo J, Cofield RH. Complications in reverse shoulder arthroplasty. EFORT Open Rev 2017;1(3):72–80
16. Sirveaux F, Favard L, Oudet D, Huquet D, Walch G, Molé D. Grammont inverted total shoulder arthroplasty in the treatment of glenohumeral osteoarthritis with massive rupture of the cuff: results of a multicentre study of 80 shoulders. J Bone Joint Surg Br 2004;86(3):388–395
17. Frankle M, Siegal S, Pupello D, Saleem A, Mighell M, Vasey M. The reverse shoulder prosthesis for glenohumeral arthritis associated with severe rotator cuff deficiency: a minimum two-year follow-up study of sixty patients. J Bone Joint Surg Am 2005;87(8):1697–1705
18. Seebauer L, Walter W, Keyl W. Reverse total shoulder arthroplasty for the treatment of defect arthropathy. Oper Orthop Traumatol 2005;17(1):1–24
19. Boileau P, Watkinson D, Hatzidakis AM, Hovorka I. Neer Award 2005: The Grammont reverse shoulder prosthesis: results in cuff tear arthritis, fracture sequelae, and revision arthroplasty. J Shoulder Elbow Surg 2006;15(5):527–540
20. Wall B, Nové-Josserand L, O'Connor DP, Edwards TB, Walch G. Reverse total shoulder arthroplasty: a review of results according to etiology. J Bone Joint Surg Am 2007;89(7):1476–1485
21. Cuff D, Pupello D, Virani N, Levy J, Frankle M. Reverse shoulder arthroplasty for the treatment of rotator cuff deficiency J Bone Joint Surg Am 2008;90(6):1244–1251
22. Cuff D, Clark R, Pupello D, Frankle M. Reverse shoulder arthroplasty for the treatment of rotator cuff deficiency: a concise follow-up, at a minimum of five years, of a previous report. J Bone Joint Surg Am 2012;94(21):1996–2000
23. Ferreira Neto AA, Malavolta EA, Assunção JH, Trindade EM, Gracitelli ME. Reverse shoulder arthroplasty: clinical results and quality of life evaluation. Rev Bras Ortop (English Edition), 2017;52(3);298–302

18 Clavicle Fracture

Matthew Baker and Uma Srikumaran

Summary

Clavicle fracture account for approximately 5% of adult fractures and there continues to be controversy in the ideal treatment.

Keywords: Clavicle fracture, collarbone, trauma

I. Epidemiology

A. Young active patients

B. Displacement:
1. Medial:
   a. Sternocleidomastoid (SCM): Pulls medial fragment posteromedially.
2. Lateral:
   a. Weight of arm and pectoralis pull lateral fragment inferomedially.
3. Open fractures → fragment buttonholes through the platysma.

C. Associated injuries are rare but include:
1. Scapulothoracic disassociation
2. Ipsilateral scapular fracture
3. Neurovascular injuries
4. Rib fracture
5. Pneumothorax
6. Lateral 1/3 fractures can have concomitant glenohumeral pathology.

II. Anatomy

A. "S" shape with six muscular attachments

B. Acts as a strut connecting the axial and appendicular skeleton

C. Sternoclavicular joint medially

D. Acromioclavicular joint laterally

E. The first bone to start ossification and the last one to complete union.

III. Classification

A. Neer:
1. Middle Third (Group 1):
   a. Nondisplaced:
      i. <100% displacement.
   b. Displaced:
      i. >100% displaced.

2. Lateral third (Group 2):
   a. Type 1:
      i. Nondisplaced
      ii. Fractures occur between the acromioclavicular (AC) and coracoclavicular (CC) ligaments and ligaments are intact
      iii. Treatment is nonoperative.
   b. Type 2:
      i. 2A:
         - CC ligaments attached to distal fragment.
      ii. 2B:
         - Trapezoid ligament intact
         - Conoid ligament torn.
      iii. Highest rate of nonunion
      iv. Consider open reduction and internal fixation (ORIF):
         - Hook plate versus ligament reconstruction with fragment fixation.
   c. Type 3:
      i. Articular fractures
      ii. Typically nondisplaced
      iii. Nonoperative treatment:
         - Distal clavicle excision for symptomatic patients.
B. Allman's classification:
   1. Distal third:
      a. Group II
      b. 15%.
   2. Middle third:
      a. Group I
      b. 80%.
   3. Medial third:
      a. Group III
      b. 5%.

IV. Imaging

A. X-rays primary imaging
B. Compare with contralateral side:
   1. Evaluate for shortening
   2. Zanca view:
      a. 15 degrees cephalad tilt.

V. Treatment

A. Nonoperative:
   1. Nondisplaced
   2. Displacement <2 cm
   3. No neurologic injury.
B. Sling versus figure of 8 brace:
   1. No difference in outcomes
   2. Patients tolerate sling immobilization more than figure of 8 bracing
   3. Range of motion (ROM) started at 2 to 4 weeks
   4. Strengthening started at 6 to 10 weeks.
C. Operative:
   1. Open fractures
   2. Vascular injury
   3. Skin tenting/compromise related to fracture displacement
   4. Floating shoulder
   5. Symptomatic malunion/nonunion.

VI. Outcomes

A. Nonoperative:
   1. Cosmetic issues with displaced fractures
   2. Nonunion:[1,2]
      a. 1–25%
      b. Risk factors: Smoking, displacement >100%, shortening >2 cm, female, advanced age, comminution, and Type II lateral 1/3 fractures.
   3. Shoulder fatigue:
      a. More than 2 cm shortening.
B. Operative:
   1. Improved functional outcomes:
      a. Especially with fractures shortened by >2 cm or displaced by 100%
      b. 88% of National football league (NFL) players after ORIF remained in the NFL 1 year after fixation.[3]
   2. Decreased time to union:
      a. 16 weeks versus 28 weeks (nonoperative).[4]
   3. Decreased symptomatic malunion rate
   4. Improved shoulder function
   5. Improved subjective shoulder function
   6. Improved cosmesis
   7. Increased risk of additional procedures
   8. Increased risk of infection.

C. Intermedullary (IM) fixation versus ORIF:
1. Much controversy regarding operative indications:
    a. IM fixation:
        i. Improved cosmesis
        ii. Lower risk of injury to the supraclavicular nerves
        iii. Increased risk of implant migration
        iv. Should not be used for comminuted or segmental fractures.
    b. ORIF:
        i. Superior plating:
            • Increased load to failure
            • Decreased deltoid detachment
            • Increased risk of neurovascular injury
            • Increased risk of hardware removal.
        ii. Anterior plating:
            • Biomechanically inferior to precontoured superior plating
            • Decreased risk of neurovascular injury and symptomatic hardware.

VII. Complications

A. Reoperation (12%)
B. Implant failure/migration:
    1. 4%.
C. Loosening of the implant:
    1. 3.2%.
D. Refracture:
    1. 1.6%.
E. Infection
F. Frozen shoulder.

Suggested Readings

Allman FL (1967). Fracture classification of the clavicle. JBJS 49A:774

Altamimi SA, McKee MD; Canadian Orthopaedic Trauma Society. Nonoperative treatment compared with plate fixation of displaced midshaft clavicular fractures: surgical technique. J Bone Joint Surg Am 2008;90(Suppl 2 Pt 1):1–8

Hyland S, Charlick M, Varacallo M. Anatomy, Shoulder and upper limb, clavicle. [Updated 2020 Apr 27]. In: StatPearls [Internet]. Treasure island (FL): StatPearls publishing; 2020 (Jan). Available from: https://www.ncbi.nlm.nih.gov/books/NBK525990/

Nourian A, Dhaliwal S, Vangala S, Vezeridis PS; Midshaft Fractures of the Clavicle. Midshaft fractures of the clavicle: a meta-analysis comparing surgical fixation using anteroinferior plating versus superior plating. J Orthop Trauma 2017;31(9):461–467

Naveen BM, Joshi GR, Harikrishnan B. Management of mid-shaft clavicular fractures: comparison between non-operative treatment and plate fixation in 60 patients. Strateg Trauma Limb Reconstr 2017;12(1):11–18

Nourian A, Dhaliwal S, Vangala S, Vezeridis PS. Midshaft fractures of the clavicle: a meta-analysis comparing surgical fixation using anteroinferior plating versus superior plating. J Orthop Trauma. 2017;31(9):461–467

Nuber GW, Bowen MK. Acromioclavicular joint injuries and distal clavicle fractures. J Am Acad Orthop Surg 1997;5(1):11–18

Paladini P, Pellegrini A, Merolla G, Campi F, Porcellini G. Treatment of clavicle fractures. Transl Med UniSa 2012;2:47–58

Ranalletta M, Rossi LA, Piuzzi NS, Bertona A, Bongiovanni SL, Maignon G. Return to sports after plate fixation of displaced midshaft clavicular fractures in athletes. Am J Sports Med 2015;43(3):565–569

Robinson CM, Court-Brown CM, McQueen MM, Wakefield AE. Estimating the risk of nonunion following non-operative treatment of a clavicular fracture. J Bone Joint Surg Am 2004;86(7):1359–1365

Robinson CM. Fractures of the clavicle in the adult: epidemiology and classification. J Bone Joint Surg Br 1998;80(3):476–484

Shin SJ, Do NH, Jang KY. Risk factors for postoperative complications of displaced clavicular midshaft fractures. J Trauma Acute Care Surg 2012;72(4):1046–1050

Van der Meijden OA, Gaskill TR, Millett PJ. Treatment of clavicle fractures: current concepts review. J Shoulder Elbow Surg 2012;21(3):423–429

Worhacz K, Nayak AN, Boudreaux RL, et al. Biomechanical analysis of superior and anterior precontoured plate fixation techniques for Neer type II-A clavicle fractures. J Orthop Trauma 2018 32(12):e462–e468

References

1. Robinson CM, Court-Brown CM, McQueen MM, Wakefield AE. Estimating the risk of nonunion following nonoperative treatment of a clavicular fracture. J Bone Joint Surg Am. 2004;86(7):1359–1365
2. Liu W, Xiao J, Ji F, Xie Y, Hao Y. Intrinsic and extrinsic risk factors for nonunion after nonoperative treatment of midshaft clavicle fractures. Orthop Traumatol Surg Res. 2015;101(2):197–200
3. Jack RA II, et al. Performance and return to sport after clavicle open reduction and internal fixation in national football league players. Orthopedic J Sports Med 2017; 5 (8)
4. Altamimi SA, McKee MD; Canadian Orthopaedic Trauma Society. Nonoperative treatment compared with plate fixation of displaced midshaft claviclar fractures: surgical technique. J Bone Joint Surg Am 2008;90(Suppl 2 Pt 1):1–8

19 Proximal Humeral Fractures

Diana Zhu and Uma Srikumaran

Summary

Proximal humeral fractures are the third most common fractures and affect both young and elderly patients. Neer's classification system is commonly used in determining fracture patterns but has recently been found to have poor reliability and reproducibility. Protecting the posterior humeral circumflex artery during fracture fixation may minimize loss of the blood supply to the humeral head as the anterolateral ascending branch of the anterior circumflex artery supplies the humeral head to a lesser degree than originally believed. Clinically significant difference in patient-reported outcomes and function have not been observed between surgical and nonoperative treatment options for proximal humeral fractures. Open reduction and internal fixation with locked plating has better functional and patient-reported outcomes than hemiarthroplasty. In the past decade, reverse shoulder arthroplasty has become an attractive approach for managing proximal humeral fractures as the prosthesis can compensate for tuberosity complications. Overall, thorough consideration of bone quality, fracture patterns, and the myriad treatment options available is necessary to successfully manage proximal humeral fractures.

Keywords: Proximal humeral fracture, open reduction and internal fixation, reverse total shoulder arthroplasty

I. Background

A. 5% of all fractures, third most common fracture

B. Female to male ratio 2–4:1

C. Increasing incidence with aging population

D. Associated injuries:
1. Nerve: Axillary
2. Vascular: Axillary (5% of four-part fractures)
3. Other: Rib fracture, pneumothorx.[1]

E. Bimodal age distribution:
1. High-energy injuries in younger patients
2. Osteoporotic fractures often associated with low-energy trauma in elderly patients.

F. Fracture patterns are dictated by bone structure and deforming muscle forces.[2]

II. Neer classification of humeral head fractures

A. Fracture defined by number of parts

B. Four parts (▶ **Fig. 19.1**):
1. Humeral head (HH)
2. Greater tuberosity (GT)

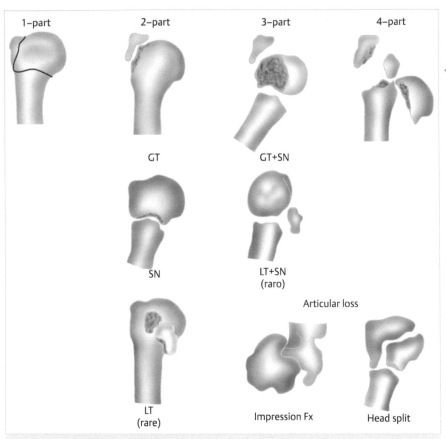

Fig. 19.1 Neer classification for proximal humeral fractures.

3. Lesser tuberosity (LT)

4. Humeral shaft (HS).

C. Definition of fracture parts:

1. Displacement >1cm, or

2. 45-degree angulation.[3]

D. Classification using the Neer system assigned on basis of computed tomography (CT) scans and radiographs are not very reliable or reproducible.[4]

III. Valgus impacted fractures (▶Fig. 19.2)

A. Not included in Neer's original classification

B. Accounts for 14 to 35% of four-part fractures

C. Preserved medial soft tissue hinge preserves blood supply to articular segment

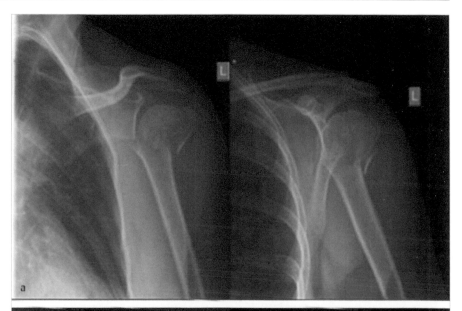

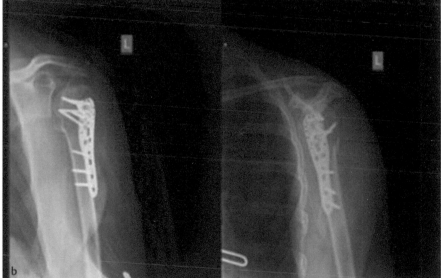

Fig. 19.2 (a, b) Valgus impacted fracture.

D. Three-part fractures:

1. Most patients treated nonoperatively report good or excellent results.[5]

E. Four-part fractures:

1. Open reduction and internal fixation (ORIF) and closed reduction percutaneous pinning (CRPP) provide satisfactory results in most patients.[6]

IV. Vascularization of the humeral head

A. Quantifying arterial vascularization of the humeral head:

1. Anterolateral ascending branch of the anterior circumflex provides 36% of the blood supply to the humeral head

2. Posterior circumflex supplies posterior portion of greater tuberosity and a small posterior inferior part of the head:

    a. Posterior humeral circumflex artery constitutes 64% of the blood supply to the humeral head.

3. Possible explanation for the relatively low rates of osteonecrosis

4. Protecting the posterior humeral circumflex artery during surgical approach may minimize loss of the blood supply to the humeral head.[7,8]

B. Humeral head ischemia and necrosis predictors:

1. There is 97% positive predictive value of ischemia if following criteria are met:

    a. Anatomic neck fracture

    b. Short calcar (<8 mm displacement)

    c. Disrupted medial hinge (>2 mm displacement).[9]

2. Using above criteria:

    a. Avascular Necrosis (AVN) group: 30% had all predictors

    b. Non-AVN group: 4.7% had all predictors.

3. The three criteria are not sufficient in determining necrosis:

    a. Recommend three-dimensional CT to better evaluate the calcar region.[10]

V. Management of proximal humeral fractures

The severity of fracture comminution and displacement may have a more significant effect on functional outcomes than the choice of treatment. There is clear difference in prognosis between three- and four-part fractures, but not between two- and three-part fractures.[11,12]

A. Nonoperative approach:

1. Entails use of sling or collar, cuff sling, and early physical therapy[13]

2. Conservative treatment of proximal humeral fractures in older patients provides adequate pain relief:

    a. However, it provides limited functional outcomes.[12]

B. ORIF:

1. Most common, often used for younger patients, and results depend on bone quality and reduction

2. Minimally invasive lateral approach is the optimal treatment for Neer's type 2 and type 3 proximal humeral fractures:

    a. Nailing provides less stability for more than two fragmented fractures.[14,15]

3. Allows for reliable fracture healing and little residual shoulder pain:[16]

    a. Mechanical failure of plates occur often due to malreduction.

4. Avoiding varus can decrease rate of postoperative failures:[17]
   a. Quantification of the deltoid muscle perfusion with dynamic contrast-enhanced ultrasound shows that benefits of the minimally invasive plate osteosynthesis approach on soft tissue might not be as beneficial as expected.[18]
5. Medial support in locked plating (▶Fig. 19.3):
   a. Evidence that medial support was established:
      i. Anatomic reduction of medial cortex
      ii. Proximal fragment impacted laterally into the distal fragment
      iii. Oblique locking screw was positioned inferomedially in the proximal head fragment.
   b. Lack of medial support resulted in:
      i. Increased loss of head height
      ii. Increased risk of penetration of screws into the articular surface
      iii. Increased loosening of screws.[19]
C. Hemiarthroplasty:
   1. Well-accepted procedure to treat four-part and three-part fractures associated with severe osteopenia, and head splitting and severe articular impression fractures

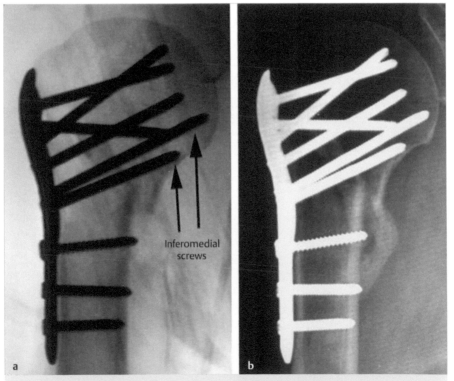

Fig. 19.3 (a, b) Medial support in open reduction and internal fixation (ORIF).

2. Satisfactory results in terms of range of motion, and pain relief can be expected in most patients.[20]

D. Closed reduction external fixation (CREF):

1. External fixation achieves safe healing and effective management for displaced proximal humeral fractures[21]

2. Percutaneous insertion of Kirschner wires from the upper lateral part of the humeral head through the medullary canal minimizes complications.[22]

E. Total shoulder arthroplasty (TSA):

1. Reduces shoulder pain effectively for acute three- and four-part proximal humeral fractures

2. Late TSA is a satisfactory reconstructive option when primary treatment of proximal humeral fractures fail.[23]

F. Reverse total shoulder arthroplasty (rTSA):

1. Attractive approach as the prosthesis can compensate for tuberosity complications[24]

2. Using a dedicated stem is a viable solution to treat complex humeral fractures as reliable restoration of elevation can be expected[25]

3. Quicker recovery but there are limited reconstructive options if complications occur

4. Use of rTSA has increased for treatment of three- and four-part proximal humeral fractures in the elderly

5. Lack of long-term studies with rTSA, so should be used conservatively for patients with high functional demands.[26-28]

VI. Comparison of approaches

A. Surgical versus nonoperative treatment:

1. Randomized controlled trials have shown no clinically important difference in patient-reported outcomes, upper-limb functions, and quality of life between two groups:[29,30]

   a. Selection bias occurs as patients are often excluded due to "clear indications for surgery."[31]

2. Fewer nonunions and complications with nonoperative treatment.[29,32]

B. Hemiarthroplasty versus rTSA:

1. rTSA shows better results than hemiarthroplasty in forward elevation, abduction; constant score; disabilities of the shoulder, arm, and hand (DASH) score; American shoulder and elbow surgeons (ASES); and tuberosity healing:

   a. No difference in external rotation.[33]

2. Since the past decade, shoulder surgeons are performing more rTSAs for proximal humeral fractures than hemiarthroplasties (HSA)[27]

3. Hemiarthroplasty has significantly fewer adverse events than rTSA

4. For three- and four-part fractures, rTSA provides significantly better functional outcomes than hemiarthroplasty.[34]

C. ORIF versus hemiarthroplasty:

    1. ORIF provides better results with three- and four-part fractures[2]

    2. Better restoration of normal anatomy with ORIF than with hemiarthroplasty:

        a. However, no difference in function with ORIF and hemiarthroplasty[35]

        b. Since 2010, shoulder surgeons are performing more rTSAs for proximal humeral fractures than HSA[27]

        c. Question still remains about ideal treatment for these fractures.

References

1. Mauro CS. Proximal humeral fractures. Curr Rev Musculoskelet Med 2011;4(4):214–220
2. Solberg BD, Moon CN, Franco DP, Paiement GD. Surgical treatment of three and four-part proximal humeral fractures. J Bone Joint Surg Am 2009;91(7):1689–1697
3. Neer CS II. Displaced proximal humeral fractures. I. Classification and evaluation. J Bone Joint Surg Am 1970;52(6):1077–1089
4. Bernstein J, Adler LM, Blank JE, Dalsey RM, Williams GR, Iannotti JP. Evaluation of the Neer system of classification of proximal humeral fractures with computerized tomographic scans and plain radiographs. J Bone Joint Surg Am 1996;78(9):1371–1375
5. Court-Brown CM, Cattermole H, McQueen MM. Impacted valgus fractures (B1.1) of the proximal humerus: the results of non-operative treatment. J Bone Joint Surg Br 2002;84(4):504–508
6. Jakob RP, Miniaci A, Anson PS, Jaberg H, Osterwalder A, Ganz R. Four-part valgus impacted fractures of the proximal humerus. J Bone Joint Surg Br 1991;73(2):295–298
7. Gerber C, Schneeberger AG, Vinh TS. The arterial vascularization of the humeral head: an anatomical study. J Bone Joint Surg Am 1990;72(10):1486–1494
8. Hettrich CM, Neviaser A, Beamer BS, Paul O, Helfet DL, Lorich DG. Locked plating of the proximal humerus using an endosteal implant. J Orthop Trauma 2012;26(4):212–215
9. Hertel R, Hempfing A, Stiehler M, Leunig M. Predictors of humeral head ischemia after intracapsular fracture of the proximal humerus. J Shoulder Elbow Surg 2004;13(4):427–433
10. Campochiaro G, Rebuzzi M, Baudi P, Catani F. Complex proximal humerus fractures: Hertel's criteria reliability to predict head necrosis. Musculoskelet Surg 2015; 99(99, Suppl 1):S9–S15
11. Hanson B, Neidenbach P, de Boer P, Stengel D. Functional outcomes after nonoperative management of fractures of the proximal humerus. J Shoulder Elbow Surg 2009;18(4):612–621
12. Torrens C, Corrales M, Vilà G, Santana F, Cáceres E. Functional and quality-of-life results of displaced and nondisplaced proximal humeral fractures treated conservatively. J Orthop Trauma 2011;25(10):581–587
13. Schumaier A, Grawe B. Proximal humerus fractures: evaluation and management in the elderly patient. Geriatr Orthop Surg Rehabil 2018;9:2151458517750516
14. Liu K, Liu PC, Liu R, Wu X. Advantage of minimally invasive lateral approach relative to conventional deltopectoral approach for treatment of proximal humerus fractures. Med Sci Monit 2015;21:496–504
15. Iacobellis C, Serafini D, Aldegheri R. PHN for treatment of proximal humerus fractures: evaluation of 80 cases. Chir Organi Mov 2009;93(2):47–56
16. Hatzidakis AM, Shevlin MJ, Fenton DL, Curran-Everett D, Nowinski RJ, Fehringer EV. Angular-stable locked intramedullary nailing of two-part surgical neck fractures of the proximal part of the humerus: a multicenter retrospective observational study. J Bone Joint Surg Am 2011;93(23):2172–2179
17. Agudelo J, Schürmann M, Stahel P, et al. Analysis of efficacy and failure in proximal humerus fractures treated with locking plates. J Orthop Trauma 2007;21(10):676–681
18. Fischer C, Frank M, Kunz P, et al. Dynamic contrast-enhanced ultrasound (CEUS) after open and minimally invasive locked plating of proximal humerus fractures. Injury 2016;47(8):1725–1731
19. Gardner MJ, Weil Y, Barker JU, Kelly BT, Helfet DL, Lorich DG. The importance of medial support in locked plating of proximal humerus fractures. J Orthop Trauma 2007;21(3):185–191
20. Hartsock LA, Estes WJ, Murray CA, Friedman RJ. Shoulder hemiarthroplasty for proximal humeral fractures. Orthop Clin North Am 1998;29(3):467–475
21. Monga P, Verma R, Sharma VK. Closed reduction and external fixation for displaced proximal humeral fractures. J Orthop Surg (Hong Kong) 2009;17(2):142–145
22. Benetos IS, Karampinas PK, Mavrogenis AF, Romoudis P, Pneumaticos SG, Vlamis J. External fixation for displaced 2-part proximal humeral fractures. Orthopedics 2012;35(12):e1732–e1737

23. Norris TR, Green A, McGuigan FX. Late prosthetic shoulder arthroplasty for displaced proximal humerus fractures. J Shoulder Elbow Surg 1995;4(4):271–280

24. Wall B, Walch G. Reverse shoulder arthroplasty for the treatment of proximal humeral fractures. Hand Clin 2007;23(4):425–430, v–vi

25. Garofalo R, Flanagin B, Castagna A, Lo EY, Krishnan SG. Reverse shoulder arthroplasty for proximal humerus fracture using a dedicated stem: radiological outcomes at a minimum 2 years of follow-up-case series. J Orthop Surg Res 2015;10(1):129

26. Gallinet D, Clappaz P, Garbuio P, Tropet Y, Obert L. Three or four parts complex proximal humerus fractures: hemiarthroplasty versus reverse prosthesis: a comparative study of 40 cases. Orthop Traumatol Surg Res 2009;95(1):48–55

27. Acevedo DC, Mann T, Abboud JA, Getz C, Baumhauer JF, Voloshin I. Reverse total shoulder arthroplasty for the treatment of proximal humeral fractures: patterns of use among newly trained orthopedic surgeons. J Shoulder Elbow Surg 2014;23(9):1363–1367

28. Gallinet D, Ohl X, Decroocq L, Dib C, Valenti P, Boileau P; French Society for Orthopaedic Surgery (SOFCOT). Is reverse total shoulder arthroplasty more effective than hemiarthroplasty for treating displaced proximal humerus fractures in older adults? A systematic review and meta-analysis. Orthop Traumatol Surg Res 2018;104(6):759–766

29. Beks RB, Ochen Y, Frima H, et al. Operative versus nonoperative treatment of proximal humeral fractures: a systematic review, meta-analysis, and comparison of observational studies and randomized controlled trials. J Shoulder Elbow Surg 2018;27(8):1526–1534

30. Handoll HH, Brorson S. Interventions for treating proximal humeral fractures in adults. Cochrane Database Syst Rev 2015; (11):CD000434

31. Ghert M, McKee M. To operate or not to operate, that is the question: the proximal humerus fracture. Bone Joint Res 2016;5(10):490–491

32. Launonen AP, Lepola V, FlinkkiLä T, Laitinen M, Paavola M, Malmivaara A. Treatment of proximal humerus fractures in the elderly: a systematic review of 409 patients. Acta Orthop 2015;86(3):280–285

33. Shukla DR, McAnany S, Kim J, Overley S, Parsons BO. Hemiarthroplasty versus reverse shoulder arthroplasty for treatment of proximal humeral fractures: a meta-analysis. J Shoulder Elbow Surg 2016;25(2):330–340

34. Mao F, Zhang DH, Peng XC, Liao Y. Comparison of surgical versus non-surgical treatment of displaced 3- and 4-part fractures of the proximal humerus: a meta-analysis. J Invest Surg 2015;28(4):215–224

35. Misra A, Kapur R, Maffulli N. Complex proximal humeral fractures in adults—a systematic review of management. Injury 2001;32(5):363–372

20 Scapular Winging

Andrew Schneider and Uma Srikumaran

Summary

This chapter presents a condensed overview of the incidence, etiology, presentation, and treatment options for medial and lateral scapular winging. Though relatively rare, undiagnosed scapular winging can have deleterious functional consequences. With timely and proper treatment, good outcomes have been reported.

Keywords: Scapular winging, shoulder, surgery, anatomy

I. General overview

A. Rare entity; incidence largely unknown due to underdiagnosis

B. Two main types of scapular winging (▶ **Fig. 20.1**):

    1. Medial scapular winging:

        a. Inferior pole of scapula translated medially and posteriorly off chest wall. Large scapular prominence can be seen on inspection.

    2. Lateral scapular winging:

        a. Inferior pole of scapula depressed and laterally shifted.

C. Caused by a dysfunction of the stabilizing muscles of the scapula, resulting in an imbalance of forces

D. Serratus anterior palsy as a result of long thoracic nerve injury is most common cause of scapular winging

E. Clinical symptoms include upper back and shoulder pain, and difficulty with overhead motion:

    1. History of trauma could indicate acute muscular detachment.

F. Treatment:

    1. Management ultimately guided by etiology of winging. Typically, nonoperative management initially for neuropraxic injuries, followed by surgical treatment if nonoperative management failed. Early surgical repair for acute muscular detachments. Trapezius palsy may benefit from early nerve procedures.

II. Anatomy

A. Stabilizing muscles:

    1. Serratus anterior:

        a. Originates from ribs 1–8

        b. Responsible for scapular protraction, holding medial border of scapula against chest wall

        c. Innervated by long thoracic nerve (C5–C7 nerve roots):

            i. Injury to this nerve causes serratus anterior palsy and results in medial scapular winging.

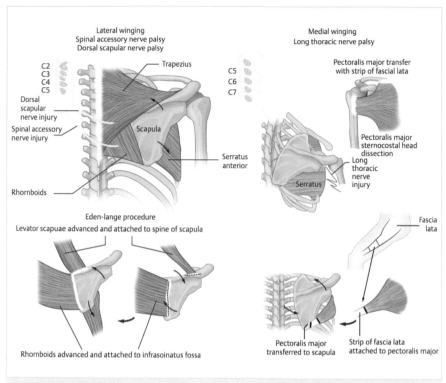

Fig. 20.1 Illustration of nerve palsies responsible for lateral and medial scapular winging, and their respective surgical treatment options.

2. Trapezius:

   a. Originates from occiput and spinous processes of C7–T12

   b. Three functional components: superior, middle, and inferior

   c. Innervated by spinal accessory nerve.

3. Rhomboid major and rhomboid minor:

   a. Rhomboid major originates from T2–T5 and inserts on medial border of scapula; rhomboid minor originates from C7–T1 and inserts on medial border of scapula just superior to rhomboid major insertion

   b. Rhomboids work together with middle portion of trapezius in scapular retraction and medial scapular border elevation

   c. Innervated by dorsal scapular nerve.

4. Levator scapulae:

   a. Originates from C1–C4 transverse processes and inserts onto medial border of scapula at the level of the scapular spine

   b. Works to elevate scapula and medially rotate its inferior angle

   c. Innervated by C3–C4, and dorsal scapular nerve.

B. Nerves:
1. Long thoracic nerve:
   a. Innervates serratus anterior
   b. Arises from anterior rami of C5–C7 nerve roots, running posterior to brachial plexus and axillary vessels
   c. Susceptible to injury by direct trauma or stretch, particularly during sports participation, due to its superficial course
   d. Can be damaged during removal of axillary lymph nodes during breast cancer surgery.
2. Spinal accessory nerve:
   a. Innervates trapezius and sternocleidomastoid muscles
   b. Cranial nerve XI: Exits skull and courses downward crossing internal jugular vein before sending branches to sternocleidomastoid and trapezius muscles.

III. Medial scapular winging

A. Deficit in serratus anterior function due to injury to the muscle itself or long thoracic nerve. Inferior pole of scapula rotated medially:
1. Most cases are result of nerve injury.
B. Pathophysiology:
1. Mechanical:
   a. Traumatic avulsion of serratus anterior
   b. Displaced fractures of the inferior pole of the scapula.
2. Neurologic:
   a. Traction injury
   b. Compression injury
   c. Direct injury.
C. Clinical presentation:
1. Blunt trauma or stretching of the nerve in athletes
2. Repetitive overhead use of arm in industrial workers
3. Penetrating trauma
4. Positioning during anesthesia
5. Viral illness.
D. Evaluation:
   a. Initial physical examination should start with full exposure of upper back to look for asymmetry in the position of the scapulae
   b. Patients will have difficulty with >120 degrees of forward flexion; end range forward flexion of arm and resisted forward flexion will increase degree of winging
   c. Pushing against wall will also magnify winging (▶ **Fig. 20.2**).

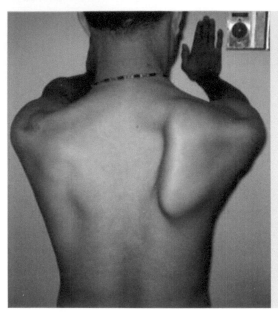

Fig. 20.2 Evaluation for serratus anterior deficit by having patient push against a wall and observing asymmetric winging of right scapula.

E. Imaging:

1. Initial workup should include shoulder and scapula X-rays:

   a. C-spine and chest X-rays may also be obtained

   b. Radiographs not usually diagnostic but can rule out fracture malunions, shoulder pathology, osteochondromas, etc. that may narrow differential diagnosis

   c. Magnetic resonance imaging (MRI) of the scapula may be helpful in the case of suspected muscular detachment.

F. Diagnostic studies:

1. Electromyography test/Nerve conduction study:

   a. Specific testing of long thoracic nerve, spinal accessory nerve, and dorsal scapular nerve can help confirm diagnosis:

      i. Obtain approximately 6 weeks after injury if still symptomatic

      ii. Repeat electromyography (EMG) at 3-month intervals can help follow return of nerve function.

   b. If EMG is normal, consider other etiologies of scapular winging.

G. Treatment:

1. Nonoperative:

   a. Physical therapy helpful for maintaining glenohumeral motion and preventing adhesive capsulitis:

      i. Range of motion exercises, periscapular muscle strengthening

      ii. Most cases resolve spontaneously over the course of about 1 year.

2. Operative: Persistent symptoms occurring >1 year are unlikely to resolve with continued conservative treatment:

    a. Tendon transfers:

        i. Many transfer procedures have been described to substitute for inadequate serratus anterior:

- Pectoralis major, pectoralis minor, clavicular or sternocostal heads of pectoralis major, teres major
- Sternocostal head of pectoralis major using fascia lata graft is most popular:
  - Lateral decubitus position
  - Sternocostal head of pectoralis major released from humerus. Graft sutured into released pectoralis major tendon and fed through drill hole in inferior angle of scapula.

    b. Scapulothoracic fusion:

        i. Large surgical undertaking with resultant significant loss of motion

       ii. Salvage procedure when other surgical treatments fail.

IV. Lateral scapular winging

A. Shoulder blade depressed, laterally translated

B. Pathophysiology:

1. Most common cause is trapezius palsy from iatrogenic spinal accessory nerve injury:

    a. Neck dissection of tumors, lymph node biopsies in posterior cervical triangle.

2. Lateral winging from rhomboid weakness secondary to dorsal scapular nerve injury is extremely rare:

    a. Entrapment and direct injuries to dorsal scapular nerve have been reported.

C. Clinical presentation:

1. May have disabling pain and muscle spasm from overcompensation of shoulder girdle muscles

2. Often have prior surgical history involving neck region.

D. Evaluation:

1. Physical examination:

    a. Trapezius wasting

    b. Unable to shrug shoulders

    c. Weakness in arm abduction, forward flexion.

2. Diagnostic studies:

    a. EMG usually confirmatory.

E. Treatment:

1. Nonoperative:

    a. Similar to initial medial winging treatment; physical therapy is helpful for maintaining glenohumeral motion and preventing adhesive capsulitis

        i. Range of motion exercises, periscapular muscle strengthening.

    b. In spinal accessory nerve lesions due to trauma, serial EMGs beginning 3 months postinjury are useful for monitoring return of nerve function.

2. Operative: Persistent symptoms occurring >1 year are unlikely to resolve with continued conservative treatment:

    a. Eden-Lange transfer:

        i. Prone or lateral decubitus positioning

        ii. Levator scapulae and rhomboids are moved laterally on the scapula (▶Fig. 20.3)

        iii. Good results, including pain relief and return of function have been reported for this procedure.

    b. Nerve procedures:

        i. Early nerve procedures such as repair, grafting, or neurolysis may be beneficial for iatrogenic or penetrating trauma to the spinal accessory nerve.

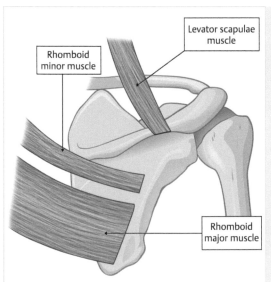

Fig. 20.3 Illustration of Eden-Lange transfer where levator scapulae and rhomboids are laterally translated on the scapula.

Suggested Readings

Gooding BW, Geoghegan JM, Wallace WA, Manning PA. Scapular winging. Shoulder Elbow 2014;6(1):4–11

Galano GJ, Bigliani LU, Ahmad CS, Levine WN. Surgical treatment of winged scapula. Clin Orthop Relat Res 2008;466(3):652–660

Martin RM, Fish DE. Scapular winging: anatomical review, diagnosis, and treatments. Curr Rev Musculoskelet Med 2008;1(1):1–11

Meininger AK, Figuerres BF, Goldberg BA. Scapular winging: an update. J Am Acad Orthop Surg 2011;19(8):453–462

Warner JJ, Navarro RA. Serratus anterior dysfunction: recognition and treatment. Clin Orthop Relat Res 1998;(349):139–148 Didesch JT, Tang P. Anatomy, etiology, and management of scapular winging. J Hand Surg Am 2019;44(4):321–330

21 Thoracic Outlet Syndrome

Alexander Bitzer and Uma Srikumaran

Summary

Thoracic outlet syndrome (TOS) refers to a group of conditions that produce varying neurologic or vascular symptoms depending on the etiology. Etiologies include compression of neurologic or vascular structures at various anatomical sites in the upper extremity with neurologic involvement being far more common. The diagnosis of thoracic outlet syndrome is largely clinical, with clinical history and physical exam findings being the most sensitive and specific. The majority of cases can be treated successfully with nonoperative management. Surgery, which aims to decompress sites of anatomic compression, may be helpful in patients with symptoms refractory to nonoperative treatment.

Keywords: Thoracic outlet syndrome, vascular, neurologic, surgery

I. General overview

A. Two separates entities:

    1. Neurogenic thoracic outlet syndrome (nTOS)

    2. Vascular thoracic outlet syndrome (vTOS).

B. Caused by anatomical sites of compression of nervous structures/brachial plexus (nTOS) or shoulder girdle vessels (vTOS)

C. Incidence is 1 to 2% of general population:

    1. nTOS is more common (19:1).

D. More common in women than men (3.5:1):

    1. Theoretical risk factors are long neck and drooping shoulders.

E. Clinical symptoms include upper extremity pain, paresthesias, numbness, weakness, fatigability, heaviness, swelling, discoloration, and Raynaud phenomenon:

    1. Pain and paresthesias most common.

F. Treatment:

    1. Operative versus nonoperative management depending on cause.

II. Anatomy

A. Nervous tissue:

    1. Brachial plexus:

        a. Five roots: C5, C6, C7, C8, T1

        b. Three trunks: Superior, middle, and inferior

        c. Six divisions: Anterior and posterior divisions of three trunks

        d. Three cords: Posterior, lateral, and medial

    e. Five branches: Median, axillary, radial, musculocutaneous, and ulnar nerves

    f. Lower trunk (C8–T1) > upper trunk (C5–C7) involvement in nTOS.

B. Vasculature:

    1. Subclavian vein:

        a. Runs anterior to interscalene triangle proximally

        b. Becomes axillary vein after crossing first rib

        c. Joins artery and brachial plexus in costoclavicular and retropectoralis minor space.

    2. Subclavian artery:

        a. Branches off brachiocephalic trunk

        b. Becomes axillary artery after crossing first rib.

    3. Axillary artery (▶ **Fig. 21.1**):

        a. Divided into three parts:

            i. First: Lateral border of first rib to superior border of pectoralis minor muscle

           ii. Second: Lies deep to the pectoralis minor muscle

          iii. Third: Extends from inferior border of the pectoralis minor muscle to the inferior border of the teres major muscle.

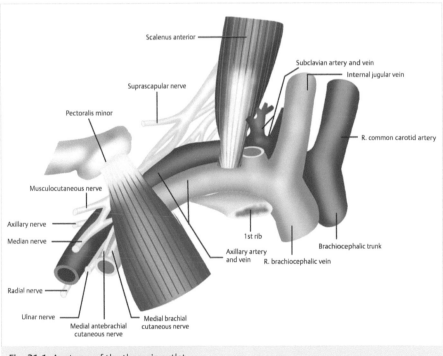

Fig. 21.1 Anatomy of the thoracic outlet.

C. Sites of compression from proximal to distal (▶ **Fig. 21.2**):

1. Interscalene triangle:
   a. Anterior scalene muscle: Anterior border
   b. Middle scalene muscle: Posterior border
   c. First rib: Inferior border.
2. Costoclavicular space:
   a. Clavicle: Anterior border
   b. First rib: Posteromedial border
   c. Costoclavicular ligament/scapula: Posterolateral border.
3. Retropectoralis minor space:
   a. Pectoralis minor: Anterior border
   b. Ribs 2 to 4: Posterior border
   c. Coracoid: Superior border.

D. Anatomical anomalies causing TOS:

1. Congenital:
   a. Soft tissue:
      i. Variation in scalene muscle origin or insertion
      ii. Presence of scalenus minimus
      iii. Fibromuscular bands constricting inlet spaces.

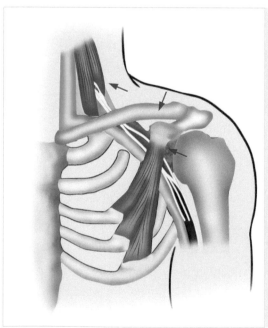

Fig. 21.2 Common sites of neurologic or vascular compression are shown. From proximal to distal, these include the interscalene triangle, the costoclavicular space, and the retropectoralis space.

b. Osseous:

    i. Presence of cervical ribs

    ii. Prominent C7 vertebrae transverse processes

    iii. First rib anomalies

    iv. Vertebral anomalies.

c. Vascular:

    i. Atypical vessel course and branching.

2. Acquired:

a. Osseous:

    i. Osteochondroma of first rib/clavicle

    ii. Malunion after fracture of first rib/clavicle

    iii. Hyperostosis

    iv. Posterior sternoclavicular dislocation.

b. Occupational:

    i. Repetitive overhead activity produces cumulative effects of micro trauma.

c. Hypertrophy:

    i. Hypertrophic scalene muscles.

III. Neurogenic thoracic outlet syndrome (nTOS)

A. Definition:

1. Compression of brachial plexus and/or distal branches

2. Lower trunk most commonly involved (C8–T1)

3. Primarily a clinical diagnosis.

B. Clinical presentation:

1. Age of onset typically between third and fifth decade of life

2. Wide variability in sensory or motor symptoms:

a. Pain, paresthesias, dysesthesia, numbness, muscle weakness, fatigability, clumsiness, and heaviness

b. Upper trunk (C5–C7):

    i. Motor: Fatigue and weakness in deltoid, biceps, and triceps

    ii. Sensory: Pain in lateral neck radiating to ear and face; follows dermatomal distributions.

c. Lower trunk (C8–T1):

    i. Motor: Fatigue and weakness in intrinsic part of hand:

      • Can lead to hand dysfunction.

    ii. Sensory: Paresthesias or dysesthesias of medial forearm, and ring and small fingers.

3. Most common complaint is pain from nerve compression
4. Pain at rest or with activity:
    a. Symptoms typically more pronounced with overhead activity and cervical rotation.
C. Evaluation:
    1. Physical examination:
        a. Neurovascular upper extremity examination:
            i. Sensation, strength, reflexes, perfusion, and pulses.
        b. Specialized tests:
            i. Adson's test:
                - Affected side: With hand on radial pulse, hyperextend shoulder/arm and have patient turn head ipsilaterally
                - Decrease in pulse amplitude + reproducibility of symptoms = positive
                - Best sensitivity of all tests along with Roos' test
                - Hoffman's test has lowest sensitivity of all tests.
            ii. Roos' test (Elevated Arm Stress Test = "EAST"):
                - With both arms at 90 degrees of abduction and external rotation, hands are slowly opened and closed for 3 minutes
                - Reproducibility of symptoms = positive.
            iii. Wright's test:
                - Affected side: Abduct and externally rotate arm as patient inhales deeply
                - Tests retropectoralis minor space
                - Best specificity of all tests.
            iv. Costoclavicular maneuver:
                - With both arms at side, retract and depress bilateral shoulders, protrude chest, and hold position
                - Pulse changes +/– reproducibility of symptoms = positive.
    2. Imaging:
        a. Cervical spine radiographs:
            i. Identify spondylosis
            ii. Identify cervical ribs
            iii. Identify clavicular or first rib abnormalities.
        b. Chest radiograph:
            i. Identify apical tumors.
        c. Computed tomography (CT)/Magnetic resonance imaging (MRI):
            i. Better visualize osseous abnormalities if necessary
            ii. Confirm space occupying lesions.

3. Diagnostic studies:
   a. Electromyography test/Nerve conduction study:
      i. Inconclusive most of the time
      ii. Difficult to interpret in double crush scenario:
         - Compression at two different sites (i.e., costoclavicular space + cubital tunnel).
      iii. Typically not sensitive enough until muscle atrophy is present.

D. Treatment:
   1. Nonoperative:
      a. Physical therapy:
         i. Work on posture:
            - Activity modification.
         ii. Strengthening of shoulder girdle muscles:
            - Trapezius, serratus anterior, levator scapulae, rhomboids, and erector spinae.
      b. Risks factors for failure of nonoperative therapy:
         i. Obesity, worker's compensation, and presence of carpal or cubital tunnel syndrome.
      c. nTOS more likely to respond to nonoperative treatment compared with vTOS
      d. Favorable response of 70% with physical therapy/exercise program
      e. Botox injections no better than placebo saline injections.
   2. Operative:
      a. Surgical treatment is performed to address the anatomical structure responsible for compression/symptoms:
         i. Scalenotomy
         ii. Scalenectomy
         iii. Cervical rib excision
         iv. First rib resection
         v. Pectoralis minor tenotomy
         vi. Claviculectomy
         vii. Supraclavicular neuroplasty.
      b. Supraclavicular or trans-axillary approach
      c. Improvement in functional and outcome scores
      d. Complication rate of 21.6% in recent systematic review
      e. More time off work required and fewer returning to work compared with nonoperative treatment
      f. No significant difference in improvement, stability, and symptom progression between operative versus nonoperative treatment in a large recent study.

IV. Vascular thoracic outlet syndrome (vTOS)

A. Definition:

1. Damage to vascular structures within the thoracic inlet

2. Caused by primary mechanical compression or thrombosis secondary to repetitive micro trauma

3. Arterial versus venous:

   a. Arterial: Subclavian artery, axillary artery

      i. First described by Wright in 1945 as due to compression of artery by pectoralis minor with arm in overhead position

      ii. Late sequelae can include intimal damage and subsequent thrombosis

      iii. Less common than venous vTOS (1:4).

   b. Venous: Subclavian vein, axillary vein:

      i. Paget-Schroetter syndrome:

         • First described as acute spontaneous venous thrombotic event

         • Recently discovered to be caused by chronic venous compressive anomaly at the thoracic outlet

         • Associated with repetitive upper extremity activities

         • Rare: 2% of all venous thromboses

         • Affects young, healthy, and athletic individuals (i.e., swimmers, weightlifters).

B. Clinical presentation:

1. Arterial:

   a. Claudication, fatigue, diminished distal upper extremity pulse, cyanosis, ischemia, night pain, and coolness.

2. Venous:

   a. Dull aching pain, venous engorgement, discoloration/mottling, and palpable axillary cord.

C. Evaluation:

1. Physical examination:

   a. Similar to nTOS with emphasis on motor function, sensation, perfusion, and pulses with subsequent changes to these with examination/specialized tests.

2. Imaging:

   a. Arteriogram/venography:

      i. Gold standard

      ii. Includes magnetic resonance angiography, computed tomography angiography, and direct catheter-based arteriography.

   b. Arterial/venous duplex ultrasound:

      i. Cost effective

      ii. Easy to obtain.

     c. Cervical spine radiographs:
         i. Evaluate osseous anomalies.
     d. Chest radiographs:
         i. Evaluate space occupying lesions.

D. Treatment:
1. vTOS typically requires a more aggressive approach compared with nTOS
2. High incidence of arterial complications when cervical ribs are present
3. Current evidence shows improved outcomes with operative treatment compared with nonoperative
4. Recent systematic review shows 90% of patients treated surgically for vTOS have excellent/good outcomes:
     a. After surgical treatment, 93% of athletes return to full competitive athletics.
5. Nonoperative:
     a. Venous:
         i. Anticoagulation
         ii. Bed rest.
     b. Arterial:
         i. Rarely indicated due to potential complications.
6. Operative:
     a. Supraclavicular or trans-axillary approach
     b. Venous:
         i. Operative intervention indicated when conservative therapy has failed
         ii. Venolysis, anticoagulation, and first rib resection
         iii. Postoperative venography:
             • Useful to confirm clot resolution
             • Dictates further need for anticoagulation.
     c. Arterial:
         i. Anticoagulation:
             • Indicated for all patients regardless of surgical intervention required.
         ii. Thrombolysis:
             • Milder cases.
         iii. Angioplasty
         iv. Thromboembolectomy:
             • More severe cases
             • Typically followed by thoracic outlet decompression.
         v. Bypass grafting
         vi. Arterial patency in >90% after thoracic outlet decompression and arterial reconstruction at 4.5 years.

Suggested Readings

Köknel Talu G. Thoracic outlet syndrome. Agri 2005;17(2):5–9 Review

Landry GJ, Moneta GL, Taylor LM Jr, Edwards JM, Porter JM. Long-term functional outcome of neurogenic thoracic outlet syndrome in surgically and conservatively treated patients. J Vasc Surg 2001;33(2):312–317, discussion 317–319

Peek J, Vos CG, Ünlü Ç, Schreve MA, van de Mortel RHW, de Vries JPM. Long-term functional outcome of surgical treatment for thoracic outlet syndrome. Diagnostics (Basel) 2018;8(1):E7

Povlsen B, Hansson T, Povlsen SD. Treatment for thoracic outlet syndrome. Cochrane Database Syst Rev 2014;(11):CD007218

Vemuri C, McLaughlin LN, Abuirqeba AA, Thompson RW. Clinical presentation and management of arterial thoracic outlet syndrome. J Vasc Surg 2017;65(5):1429–1439 Rayan GM. Thoracic outlet syndrome. J Shoulder Elbow Surg 1998;7(4):440–451 Review

22 Perioperative Pain Management for Shoulder Surgery

Ian S. Patten and Uma Srikumaran

Summary

Adequate management of pain after shoulder surgery is paramount to post-operative recovery. Regional anesthesia has proven to provide superior pain control and recovery. Several brachial plexus blocks have been described with intrascalene being the most common employed. A full knowledge of anatomy as well as the indications and potential complications associated with regional anesthesia is required by the physician.

Keywords: Pain management, peripheral nerve blocks, intrascalene, supraclavicular

I. General overview

A. First peripheral block was performed by William Halsted with cocaine in 1885

B. Over the past 30 years there has been an increasing trend in the use of peripheral nerve blocks for postoperative pain management

C. Adequate pain control via peripheral block:

1. Decreases hospital length of stay

2. Allows transition from traditional inpatient surgery to outpatient

3. Decrease opioid use and associated opioid side effects

4. Enhances participation in rehabilitation

5. Improve functions and patient satisfaction outcomes

6. Enhance cost-effectiveness.

D. Vital to understand the indications and potential complications associated with regional anesthesia.

II. Anatomy

A. Brachial plexus (▶ **Fig. 22.1**):

1. Five roots: C5, C6, C7, C8, and T1

    a. Level of intrascalene block.

2. Three trunks: Upper, middle, and lower

    a. Level of supraclavicular block.

3. Six divisions: Anterior and posterior divisions of three trunks

4. Three cords: Posterior, lateral, and medial

    a. Level of intraclavicular block.

5. Five branches: Median, axillary, radial, musculocutaneous, and ulnar nerves

    a. Level of axillary block.

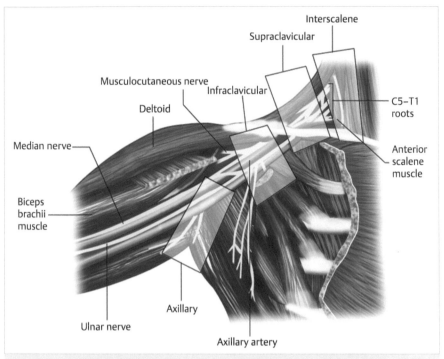

Fig. 22.1 Brachial plexus anatomy. Areas within borders represent anatomic locations of common regional blocks for upper extremity surgery. From proximal to distal: interscalene, supraclavicular, infraclavicular, and axillary.

B. Shoulder sensory innervation:

  1. Superior region:

    a. Superficial cervical plexus (C3–C4):

      i. Supraclavicular nerve.

  2. Axillary region:

    a. T2 nerve root.

  3. Shoulder capsule, subacromial bursa, acromioclavicular joint, cutaneous tissue:

    a. Suprascapular nerve—primarily C5, C6 with some C4.

C. Four anatomic regions pertinent to peripheral nerve blocks (▶ **Fig. 22.2**):

  1. Intrascalene:

    a. Potential space between anterior and middle scalenes

    b. Targets brachial plexus at root-trunk level

    c. Most commonly preformed

    d. Effective for shoulder, proximal humerus, and distal clavicle

    e. Ulnar sparing:

      i. C8 frequently not covered

      ii. Additional block required for surgery around the elbow.

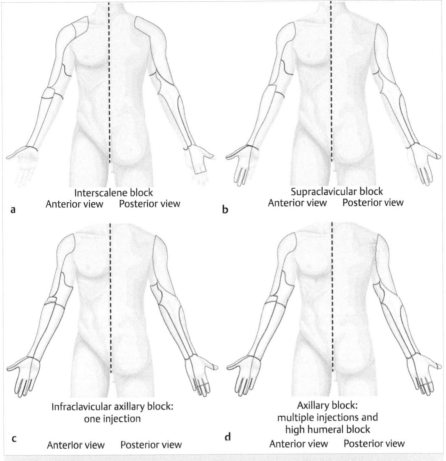

Fig. 22.2 Anterior and posterior distribution of common regional blocks. (a) Interscalene. (b) Supraclavicular. (c) Infraclavicular. (d) Axillary.

2. Supraclavicular:

   a. Superior to clavicle at the level of plexus trunks

   b. Between anterior and middle scalenes at the first rib

   c. Apical lung vulnerable

   d. Suitable for shoulder; theoretically does not cover superior aspect of shoulder, arm, and elbow: forearm hand adequately covered.

3. Infraclavicular:

   a. Boarders consist of:

      i. Superior—posterior aspect of clavicle

      ii. Inferior—soft tissues of axilla

      iii. Anterior—pectoralis minor

      iv. Posterior subscapularis.

       b.   Level of the cords before axillary and musculocutaneous nerves exit

       c.   Shoulder not covered; arm, elbow, and forearm hand adequately covered.

  4.   Axillary and suprascapular:

       a.   In combination similar shoulder coverage compared with intrascalene block

       b.   Axillary:

          i.   Located beneath glenohumeral joint between the chest wall and medial upper arm

         ii.   In isolation may be adequate for elbow surgery.

       c.   Suprascapular:

          i.   Level of the suprascapular notch.

III. Regional anesthesia

A. Definition:

  1.   Administration of local anesthetics to an area resulting in motor and sensory blockade

  2.   Central versus peripheral blocks depend on distance from spinal cord.

B. Peripheral nerve block should be conducted in awake patients:

  1.   Allow for real-time feedback from patient and avoidance of complications

  2.   Supported by level 1 evidence.

C. Localization techniques:

  1.   Ultrasound:

       a.   Faster block onset and improved success versus peripheral nerve stimulator

       b.   Less risk of vascular puncture.

  2.   Peripheral nerve stimulator:

       a.   Low intensity, short-duration electrical stimulus

       b.   Obtain a response (twitch or sensation) to localize peripheral nerve.

  3.   Needle guidance:

       a.   First methods based on anatomical landmarks and elicitation of paresthesias as the needle was advanced through the sheath.

D. Single injection versus continuous catheter:

  1.   Single injection:

       a.   Duration varies from 2 to 48 hours, average 12 hours.

  2.   Continuous catheter:

       a.   Continuous anesthesia providing relief beyond 12 hours

       b.   Patients discharged home with "pump"

    c. Studies demonstrated decreased opioid use, improved pain scores, and improved sleep patterns with use

    d. Technically more difficult

    e. Concern for toxic volume of anesthetic.

IV. Patient factors to consider

A. Obesity:
1. Patients with body mass index (BMI) >30 are 1.62 times more likely to have a failed block.

B. Use of systemic anticoagulation:
1. American Society of Regional Anesthesia and Pain Medicine consensus statement—patients who are mildly anticoagulated are safe to undergo block
2. International normalized ratio (INR) <3 noted to have 3 months bleeding risk of 3%. Increased to 7% with INR over 4.

C. Pulmonary disease:
1. Relative contraindication to proximal blocks
2. Concern in patients with poor respiratory reserve due to long-term phrenic nerve injury caused by intraneural injection, trauma, or toxicity
3. Using ultrasound and low volume have been recently shown to be safe:
    a. A randomized clinical trial that compared ultrasound-guided injections of ropivacaine, 20 mL and 5 mL, found that patients who received the low volume injection had significantly less respiratory compromise without a significant difference in pain score, opioid consumption, or sleep quality 24 hours after surgery.
4. Consider axillary and supraclavicular block versus intrascalene or supraclavicular to avoid risk of injury to apical lung or phrenic nerve compromise.

V. Medications

A. Block agents:
1. Administration:
    a. Dose dependent on agent used, technique, and preference of physician.
2. Long-acting agents:
    a. Bupivacaine:
        i. Local anesthetic
        ii. Associated with life-threatening cardiotoxicity and neurotoxicity secondary to stereospecificity to receptors.
    b. Levobupivacaine and ropivacaine:
        i. Optically pure isomer
        ii. Less neurotoxicity and cardiotoxicity compared with bupivacaine
        iii. No significant difference in efficacy.

B. Adjuvants:
    1. Epinephrine:
        a. Decreases systemic absorption
        b. Potential increased uptake by nerve
        c. Possible risk of bradycardic and hypotensive episodes
        d. Potential for allergy.
    2. Clonidine:
        a. Alpha 2 adrenergic agonist
        b. Improves effectiveness of local anesthetic
        c. Independently acts as analgesic
        d. Potential for rebound hypotension.
    3. Dexamethasone:
        a. Increases duration of sensory blockade
        b. Mechanism not well understood
        c. Has been shown in randomized trial of shoulder surgery to increase duration of sensory block and decrease opioid use.

VI. Complications

A. Systemic:
    1. Major:
        a. Cardiac arrest
        b. Respiratory failure
        c. Seizures
        d. Death.
    2. Minor:
        a. Agitation, anxiety
        b. Visual disturbances
        c. Perioral anesthesia
        d. Dizziness
        e. Muscle fibrillation
        f. Tinnitus.
    3. Incidence reported to be less than 1 in 1,000
    4. No reported cases of death attributed to peripheral block with ropivacaine or levobupivacaine
    5. Possible role for intralipid infusion to manage cardiac toxicity

6. Patients in beach chair position may be more prone to bradycardia and hypotension:

    a. Mediated by Bezold-Jarisch reflex:

        i. Venous pooling caused by seated position increases sympathetic tone resulting in a low-volume hypercontractile ventricle

        ii. May be aggravated by epinephrine.

B. Nerve injury:

    1. Relatively rare, approximately 0.4 per 1,000 blocks

    2. Paresthesias during block placement have a higher association with postoperative neurological symptoms.

C. Pneumothorax:

    1. Most common with supraclavicular block

    2. Decreased risk with use of ultrasound guidance.

Suggested Readings

Bruce BG, Green A, Blaine TA, Wesner LV. Brachial plexus blocks for upper extremity orthopaedic surgery. J Am Acad Orthop Surg 2012;20(1):38–47

Hughes MS, Matava MJ, Wright RW, Brophy RH, Smith MV. Interscalene brachial plexus block for arthroscopic shoulder surgery: a systematic review. J Bone Joint Surg Am 2013;95(14):1318–1324

Hussain N, Goldar G, Ragina N, Banfield L, Laffey JG, Abdallah FW. Suprascapular and interscalene nerve block for shoulder surgery: a systematic review and meta-analysis. Anesthesiology 2017;127(6):998–1013

Mian A, Chaudhry I, Huang R, Rizk E, Tubbs RS, Loukas M. Brachial plexus anesthesia: a review of the relevant anatomy, complications, and anatomical variations. Clin Anat 2014;27(2):210–221 Review

Review Srikumaran U, Stein BE, Tan EW, Freehill MT, Wilckens JH. Upper-extremity peripheral nerve blocks in the perioperative pain management of orthopaedic patients: AAOS exhibit selection. J Bone Joint Surg Am. 2013;95(24):e197(1-13)

Index